Praise for

TDOS Solution

"Peter Greenlaw is not a doctor; this is his strength, since he can enjoy the freedom and the courage to write what doctors are afraid to write and to say what doctors don't tell you. In this book he highlights the four points that prevent us from living long healthy lives—points that have been neglected for too long. He dissects the problems, he proposes the solutions. This book has its place among the most interesting writing of the past few years, and it should sit in the library of all those interested in knowing the truth beyond what doctors and media representatives tell us. Its place is right next to the books of Nobel Laureate Kary Mullis, University Professor Henry Bauer, Canadian Mathematician Rebecca Culshaw, and British Journalist Joan Shenton."

—MARCO RUGGIERO, MD, PHD
Retired Professor of Molecular Biology at the University of Firenze, Italy

"I congratulate the authors for bringing to light the major problems associated with our ever more increasingly toxic environment and greater nutritional deficiencies, obesity, and stress. I have come to know that the co-factors creating the TDOS Syndrome have become the most destructive component of our health. Peter Greenlaw, Dr. Messina, and Drew Greenlaw have provided a marvelous gift to the reader to enable them to understand the problem of the TDOS Syndrome in their first book. And they now present in *TDOS Solutions* what needs to be done to correct this.

Finally we have a way to help our bodies to work the way nature intended. This book will give you the knowledge and desire to finally become healthy and to also rid yourselves of excess fat that will make you feel so much better."

—DR. DENNIS HARPER
Dr. Harper, now retired, was in a general medical practice for 20 years, with 16 years devoted to the practice of complementary medicine. He was one of three people that advocated the DSHEA (Dietary Supplement

Health and Education Act) initiated under Senator Hatch. The act saved the health food industry from overregulation by the FDA. Before his retirement Dr. Harper held many offices and memberships, including as voting member of the American Osteopathic Association, President of Physicians for Progressive Medicine, Second Vice President of the Utah Osteopathic Association, Member of the Unproven Medical Procedures Committee at the Utah Medical Association, Chairman at the licensing board of the state of Utah, and fellow of the Federation of State Medical Boards.

Dr. Harper is the author of *Cleansing for Life: Nature's Best Kept Health Secret.*

TDOS
Solutions

THE GREENLAW REPORT SERIES

The TDOS Syndrome
When Toxicity, Nutritional Deficiency, Overweight, and Stress (TDOS) Collide to Threaten Our Health

TDOS Solutions
Fighting Toxicity, Nutritional Deficiency, Overweight, and Stress Syndrome (TDOS)

TDOS
Solutions

Fighting Toxicity, Nutritional Deficiency,
Overweight, and Stress Syndrome (TDOS)

Peter Greenlaw

WITH NICHOLAS MESSINA, MD, AND DREW GREENLAW

SelectBooks, Inc.
New York

The TDOS Syndrome® is a trademark of Peter Greenlaw.

Copyright © 2017 by Peter Greenlaw

This edition published by SelectBooks, Inc.
For information address SelectBooks, Inc., New York, New York.

First Edition

ISBN 978-1-59079-411-1

Library of Congress Cataloging-in-Publication Data

Names: Greenlaw, Peter, author.| Messina, Nicholas, author.
Title: TDOS solutions : fighting toxicity, nutritional deficiency, overweight, and stress (TDOS) syndrome/ Peter Greenlaw, with Nicholas Messina, MD.
Description: First edition.| New York : SelectBooks, Inc., [2017]| Series:

The Greenlaw report series| Includes bibliographical references and index.
Identifiers: LCCN 2016052224| ISBN 9781590794111 (paperback)
Subjects: LCSH: Environmental toxicology.| Environmental health.| Solutions.
Classification: LCC RA1226 .G73 2017| DDC 615.9/02--dc23 LC record available at https://lccn.loc.gov/2016052224

Book design by Janice Benight

Manufactured in the United States of America
10 9 8 7 6 5 4 3 2 1

Contents

Foreword

Catherine E. Hylwa, MD

We often hear some version of the saying that admitting there is a problem is the first step to solving it. But what about the next steps? What about getting to the solution? I am excited to say that I have discovered a way, and you can, too!

Mr. Peter Greenlaw is a renowned health and wellness expert. As a contributor to the *New Health Conversation*™ *TV program* and his new TV program and book series, *The Greenlaw Report*™, and more than a decade of studying toxins and their effects on our lives, he is in a unique position to offer alternatives to leading unhealthy nutritional lifestyles. Mr. Greenlaw has given more than 1,200 lectures worldwide and tells his audiences that they have been granted a "do-over," a second chance to a healthier life. By paying attention to necessary changes in their lives, they will be able to maximize their wellness potential. He reveals how each of us can use this knowledge to take back our lives and get the most from the second chance we have been given. He helps us identify the problems and offers solutions.

I have been fortunate to have heard Mr. Greenlaw speak on numerous occasions, and I am always inspired by his passion, his knowledge, and his commitment to better the world. He engages his audience, moving up the aisles to interact with everyone, even the back row! His journey serves as an example to us all. If you leave one of his talks and are not moved to action, then you weren't listening!

In his book *The TDOS Syndrome*, Mr. Greenlaw showed us the universal problem. Four co-factors conspire against our health and wellness plans on a daily basis: Toxicity, nutritional Deficiency, Overweight, and Stress. We need to be constantly aware of these, every day.

In this book, *TDOS Solutions*, he gives us the tools necessary to fight back! We learn ways to attack toxins with a multifaceted approach. We use nutrition containing the right proteins, along with aloe vera, enzymes, prebiotic fiber, amino acids, and good fats. We combat nutritional deficiencies by including "the mineral suite" of macro and micro minerals essential to rebuild our bodies. We replace what we have been missing with botanicals, vitamins, and nutrients. We tackle overweight issues with a low-calorie, *nutrient-dense* intake and intermittent cleanse/fasting days to help decrease cravings and prevent hunger. Finally, we are able to confront stress head on and take away its power with proper hydration, exercise, meditation, and the recognition of our "relaxation signature."

I personally have adopted the nutritional protocols outlined in this book and have increased my productivity and focus exponentially! I tell everyone I know that I have regained two useful hours a day because of this program. Time has the value of gold in a doctor's life. Not only have I received the gifts of time and energy back, but, more important, I have been given the solutions to share with others. I discuss the TDOS Syndrome with my patients and friends to help them make important health choices that best suit their needs. My husband and fellow physician in practice has also made life changes for himself and his patients. There are many of us who are walking testimonies to the power of great nutrition. As a practicing physician and wellness advocate, I feel strongly that the people in my care have benefited from what I have discovered and shared. I have always believed that it is my responsibility to give my patients the best information I can to assist them in living their lives to the fullest. *TDOS Solutions* is an outstanding source for this information.

I taught at a residency program early in my medical career, and the residents always complained about having too much work and too little time. Come to think of it, we complained of the same thing when I was a resident. If only we had all known about *TDOS Solutions*, then. We knew the problem; now we know the solution!

—Catherine E. Hylwa, MD
Diplomate of the American Board of Internal Medicine
Practicing Internist and Wellness Advocate

Acknowledgments

I want to thank my agent Bill Gladstone and Waterside Productions for believing in us in the first place.

Special thanks to the many researchers who contributed invaluable information to this book.

To our coauthor, Nicholas Messina MD, who without his encouragement, great perspective, insight, and research, this book might never have come to light.

Thanks to Michelle Kriegel for her contributions to this book.

We owe a considerable debt of gratitude to John for all of his knowledge and discoveries that led us to the new frontiers of nutritional science.

Thank you to Randall Fitzgerald for your incredible guidance that so enhanced this book.

I want to express great gratitude to my family, including my wife Sarah, who was there from our very first book with unconditional love and support.

A special thank you to my youngest son, Colin, who has been a great advocate for the discoveries that we have made and is living proof that there is hope for the next generations.

And also to my oldest son, Drew, as the coauthor and tireless worker to bring this book to life.

And thank you to my wonderful publisher SelectBooks, who believed in our work and brought this message to the world.

A Note to the Reader

The content of my book *TDOS Solutions* is not intended to diagnose, treat, or cure any diseases or to be a substitute for proven medical advice, treatments, protocols, or prescription drug therapies. None of these statements have been evaluated by the FDA. It is always recommended to check with your health professional before embarking on any diet, exercise, or nutritional plan.

It is important to note that the authors of this book receive no financial compensation from any of The Solution Providers presented in this book. We will be continually adding new solutions and Solution Providers to www.TheGreenlawReport.com. Please feel free to check in from time to time to see any new additions made to the website.

Introduction

TDOS Solutions Overview

We need a new approach to health, as my first book, *The TDOS Syndrome*, hopefully made clear. The reason is simple: The basic rules for getting healthy and staying healthy have changed. Whether it's about removing toxins, excess pounds, and stress from our bodies, or absorbing necessary nutrients, it's time to view and treat the human body as a whole system, and not merely a collection of constituent parts.

Weight loss, for example, can no longer be viewed as simply a process of losing pounds, and the techniques can't only be targeted towards shrinking the waistline. The body is a system, and it only makes sense to treat it accordingly, with solutions that are holistic and synergistic.

The TDOS Syndrome book was introduced to you as the collaboration of four co-factors that individually are capable of causing any number of health problems. But when they synthesize and synergize with one another, the problems grow increasingly dangerous, as we documented in book one.

Much in the same way I discovered what I termed "the TDOS Syndrome®," my coauthors and I have developed what we believe constitutes the most effective, multi-faceted approach that you can use to manage these problems: "the TDOS Solution."

I did not discover the TDOS Syndrome or TDOS Solutions for the reasons that most would expect. I have no formal education in medicine, science, or nutrition. I am not a doctor and this has proven to be advantageous to me. It has allowed me a unique perspective when studying the varying opinions and research and cherry picking only the best of the best from everywhere. With that being said, I mean no disrespect to all the amazing physicians and researchers out there; in fact, I have been fortunate to learn and study under some of the leading doctors, researchers and scientists from across the globe, all of which are at the top of their fields of expertise. I found my way into this field because of my own personal health struggles.

After an annual visit to my general physician almost two decades ago, it became clear in that moment that I needed to make some drastic health changes. I took my diagnosis to heart and went out to find the best ways to alleviate my health concerns, which I did. As I continued down the research rabbit hole, after reading hundreds of books, attending lectures and compiling all this incredible information it only made sense to share my findings with the world. Since then, I have been blessed to speak all over the world, giving well over 1,000 lectures, sharing my latest findings in hopes of improving the quality of life of anyone that hopefully hears my message. I feel privileged to have been given the nickname of "The Researcher of Researchers" by some of my mentors and heroes in the world of health and wellness; and I believe that is who I am.

Exactly how can we take each co-factor and either eliminate it, or reduce its influence on our ability to maximize our quality of life potential? These answers will present themselves in the remaining pages of this book.

We will reveal a revolutionary nutritional technology and its application to reduce your toxic load and your waistline, an approach that changed my life and can change the lives of countless others. It will underscore our contention that reducing calories and performing exercise isn't the most effective way to lose weight and keep it off in the twenty-first century.

Please know that I am not suggesting there is a "one size fits all" program for you. But, rather, there are a variety of excellent options for you to consider and combine together, adapting them to your own body, lifestyle, and personal needs.

The first essential step is for each of us to commit to becoming responsible for our own health and safety. We have one body to last us a lifetime; there are no spares.

My coauthors and I invite you to consider the information offered in this book and make your own decisions. If you choose to take on the challenges and techniques and follow our recommendations, you may increase the odds of living healthier—and longer—while maximizing your potential for a high quality of life.

"Any sustainable change from the status quo must start from a grassroots level. In order to change unhealthy lifestyles, which lead to disease, people need to have skin in the game. 'Band-Aid medicine' creates a false sense of security, complacency, and inhibits acceptance of personal responsibility for one's health. If good choices and behaviors within the health-care system were coupled with financial incentives, and bad choices and behaviors were coupled with financial disincentives, perhaps leverage for change would be created."

—NICHOLAS MESSINA, MD

WHY THE TDOS SOLUTIONS WILL IMPROVE YOUR HEALTH

- **Liver Support**–The liver is the main detoxifying organ of the body. It stores fat-soluble toxins so that they can be excreted in the urine. This is made easier with the amino acids in the products recommended in this book.

- **Antioxidant Protection**–Free radicals damage cells. Antioxidants are substances that fight free radicals and they are part of the TDOS Solutions.

- **Weight Loss**–It's proven that weight loss decreases the chances of diabetes, cancer, and heart disease, thus increasing your life expectancy, and following the TDOS Solutions leads to weight loss.

- **Enhanced Mental Abilities**–A recent study revealed that mental abilities improve with weight loss. Many TDOS Solution users report weight loss as a benefit and therefore improved concentration and focus.

- **Increased Energy**–Do you want to feel better and accomplish more? The TDOS Solution isn't an "energy drink," but rather delivers a level of nutrition that will help you achieve more each day without feeling like you have been overworked.

- **Immune Support**–Nutritional fasting (one of the key TDOS Solutions) and removing impurities from the body, while replenishing it with vital nutrients, can improve immune function and lessen immunity threats within the body.

- **Better Cellular Function**–Our cells need essential nutrients and compounds to be healthy and communicate. Nutritional fasting delivers such nutrients and creates an environment where cells can effectively communicate and perform.

- **Premature-Aging Protection**–Nutrient deficiencies, impurities, and toxins can damage our cells and organs and lead to premature aging. Nutritional fasting slows the onslaught of the toxic world and creates a shield of protection for increased energy and a sense of overall rejuvenation.

- **Better Digestion**–The TDOS Solution products deliver enzymes and other vital nutrients for the digestive tract. The digestive system is replenished with good bacteria and enzymes to help with the breakdown and absorption of food.

- **Enhanced Nutrition**–The best way to take control of your health is through improved nutrition. One of the few things in life that you can control is what goes into your body–and what goes into your body determines what type of body you will have. *TDOS Solutions* offers a terrific new nutritional approach.

- **Weight Control**–It's no secret that weight control is a huge problem in today's society. Nutritional fasting may help support the loss of excess fat and water and increase muscle mass, keeping weight stabilized and avoiding weight gain.

- **Fighting Obesity**–Obesity is on the rise and has been rising since 1985 when the CDC (Center for Disease

Control and Prevention) started to monitor obesity. Many degenerative diseases are associated with obesity, either as the cause or a complicating factor. Nutritional fasting as part of a healthy lifestyle can be a weapon in the fight against obesity.

- **Adaptogenic Support**–Some of the approaches in *TDOS Solutions* contain adaptogens, which have been used by Olympic athletes for years. Adaptogens are agents (usually botanicals) that help the body "adapt" to physical and mental stress.

- **Less food Cravings**–As you nutritionally fast it's very common to have cravings for unhealthy foods disappear. These cravings are replaced with a sense of well-being and satiety.

- **An "Aura" of Wellness**–Want to look good and have that air of good health and energy? It's almost impossible to do this if you're not eating nutritionally dense foods like those from *TDOS Solutions*.

- **Youthful Skin**–Skin cannot be healthy without the proper nutrition from the inside. This also applies for impurities in the body. Nutritional fasting and replenishing your body with vital nutrients can lead to smooth, youthful-looking skin.

- **Rejuvenation with "Mineral Suites"**–The *TDOS Solutions* approach contains vitamins, nutrients, and essential major minerals (macro minerals), essential trace (micro) minerals and trace elements, which are the key to a healthy body. Cells cannot function properly without them. Minerals and trace elements are easily absorbed and, once in the body, speed up innumerable cellular reactions.

- **Gastrointestinal Health Support**–Replacing poor-quality, low-fiber foods with high-quality, nutritionally dense foods can improve digestion and enhance gastro-intestinal function.

- **Solution Providers**–For your convenience we provide suggestions for TDOS Solution Providers that you can go directly to for additional support. These Solution Providers can provide additional information and protocols that can help you to maximize your quality of life potential. Of course, you are free to seek out your own Solution Providers utilizing the guidelines for what to look for that we have laid out in this book.

PART ONE

Problems Identified, Problems Solved

Chapter One

Toxicity Interventions

The following is a summary of the problem of toxicity (as identified in our book *The TDOS Syndrome*)

- We each carry a "body burden" of hundreds, if not thousands, of synthetic chemicals that persist in our body fat, absorbed from contact with food, water, air, consumer products, and industrial processes, that accumulate over a lifetime. Because toxins migrate, their molecules attached to dust particles blowing in the wind, no one can escape them anywhere on the planet.

- These potentially toxic chemicals can interact synergistically inside of us, producing a range of possible negative health effects. Many of the health effects haven't been adequately identified or studied yet.

- Even low-dose chemical exposures, at what were once thought to be safe levels, can still affect the hormonal systems of the human body.

- Some low-dose chemicals, nontoxic on their own, become toxic and cancer-causing when mixed with other seemingly safe chemicals.

- Even before birth, we absorb and inherit chemicals directly from our mothers, based on their chemical exposure. These contaminants and their toxic effects can persist throughout a lifetime.

- Because our food supply has become nutritionally bank-rupt, we lack sufficient nutrition for the body to have the fuel it so desperately needs to energize the immune system and our toxin-cleansing organs, in order to com-bat this onslaught of toxicity.

- Some types of hormone-disrupting toxins in our bodies, called obesogens, can trigger weight gain. This interaction between toxins and fat cells is one of the scientifical-ly documented, but rarely recognized, reasons behind the overweight and obesity epidemic in the US and the world.

- Toxins are playing a major role in the breakdown of the body's functions, particularly in undermining the liver's effectiveness as a toxin remover. Until we reduce their numbers, in terms of exposure to them and in terms of their presence inside of us, the negative health symp-toms resulting from toxins will continue. Although we are living longer, we are living sicker.

ANTIDOTES TO THE "BODY BURDEN"

To measure how much of a body burden of toxins he had absorbed over a lifetime, and whether a detoxification program could help reduce those toxin levels, a middle-aged investigative reporter had his blood tested. Then he entered a health facility to undergo its detox regimen.

Of the few dozen chemicals, he was tested for by a toxicology lab in Dallas, using eight vials of his blood and a urine sample, results indicated a slew of them in his body fat and blood, all at elevated levels usually considered "abnormal."

Among the chemicals found in him were the pesticides DDE, HCB, and Mirex. Among the heavy metals was arsenic. Fire-retardant chemicals showed up, as did a range of chemicals from consumer products. Nearly every chemical the lab tested him for was found at some level in his blood.

It's important to note that toxin levels found in the blood don't adequately reveal the true extent of a person's toxicity. Toxicologists point out that if a blood test detects four parts per billion molecules of a toxin that really means the body fat could contain 800 parts per billion, or more, depending on the chemical and where it is stored in the body. A measuring ratio of about one to four is used when it comes to levels in the blood versus body fat levels.

Immediately after receiving his lab results, the reporter checked himself into a three-week program at the Hippocrates Health Institute in West Palm Beach, Florida. This facility offers a raw vegan foods diet, wheatgrass juice (which is high in chlorophyll), and green plant juices, as the basis for reinvigorating the immune system to combat illness and disease.

The detox part of this regimen involved supplementing the nutrient-dense living foods diet with periodic intermittent nutritional fasting, vigorous exercise followed by the use of a far infrared sauna every day, colon cleanses, and ingesting chlorella tablets (a green algae-based supplement). Also, no synthetic chemicals are allowed at the facility, which excludes most personal care products, cosmetics, sunscreens, and the like, to keep further body absorption of chemicals to a minimum.

After just four days on the program, the reporter had lost 10 pounds. He also noted how he felt invigorated, with a high-energy level, despite being in withdrawal from caffeine, which isn't allowed at Hippocrates. At the end of three weeks, he had his blood and urine samples sent to the same toxicology lab in Dallas and re-tested. When the results came back, lab director and biochemist Dr. John Laseter phoned the journalist, Randall Fitzgerald.

"Your detox had an impact," marveled Dr. Laseter. "Your total chemical load dropped out of the picture."

Most of the toxins detected in Fitzgerald's blood before entering the detox program had reached almost undetectable levels after the three-week detox. Fitzgerald chronicled his detox experience in his 2006 book, *The Hundred Year Lie: How to Protect Yourself from the Chemicals That Are Destroying Your Health.*

This journalist's experience demonstrated that we can effectively summon outside defenses against the chemical onslaught. We can detoxify our bodies and, in the process, protect ourselves against the TDOS Syndrome.

USE FAR-INFRARED SAUNAS
FOR DETOXIFICATION

Far Infrared is produced by the sun as a band of light that cannot be seen but can be felt as heat. It is the heat you feel on a cold day when the sun warms your skin.

This energy is absorbed by the body and gently elevates the body's core temperature a few degrees. A sauna using this method has infrared heaters emitting the light, which is absorbed by the surface of the user's skin. Far Infrared saunas penetrate the skin into body tissues at a much deeper level than do ordinary steam saunas.

Through a process called resonant absorption, Far Infrared removes toxins out of the body's fat cells via perspiration, respiration, urine, and stool. Being able to remove toxins out of fat cells is important because that is where toxins are stored when toxic exposure exceeds the body's natural ability to remove them.

Analysis of sweat, urine, and stool after exposure to a Far Infrared Sauna Therapy shows the excretion of pesticides, chemicals, environmental poisons, carcinogens, endocrine disruptors, obesogens, and heavy metals, such as lead, mercury, cadmium, arsenic, aluminum, chromium, copper, and nickel.

A September 2011 study in the science journal *Alternative Medicine Review* noted how "studies document the effectiveness of sauna therapy for persons with hypertension, congestive heart failure, and for post-myocardial infarction (heart attack) care. Some individuals with chronic obstructive pulmonary disease, chronic fatigue, chronic pain, or addictions also find benefit."

The study review continued: "Overall, regular sauna therapy (either radiant heat or far-infrared units) appears to be safe and offers multiple health benefits to regular users {including} existing evidence that supports the use of saunas as a component of purification or cleansing protocols for environmentally induced illness,"[1] which is to say, exposure to, and the absorption of, toxins.

Far-Infrared and Its impact on Weight Management

According to Dr. Sherry Rogers, in her book *It's Not Your Fault You're Fat*, "Permanent weight loss begins by getting the damaging toxins out of the body. You see, we are the first generation ever exposed to thousands of environmental toxins every day in our air, food and water. These toxins are unavoidable, and when they surpass the ability of the body to detoxify them, we silently, yet steadily, tank up on them." Toxins can cause obesity and also induce health problems associated with obesity, such as inflammation, insulin resistance, and oxidative stress, inability to regulate appetite, altered thyroid metabolism, cancer, and diabetes.

BPA, a fundamental component in plastics, is an endocrine disruptor that is stored in fat cells and is extremely difficult to remove from the body. The accumulation of BPA in fat is three times higher than in other tissues. BPA harms reproductive organ function, causes neurological impairment, and places the body at a high risk for breast and prostate cancer. BPA programs fat cells to incorporate more fat and results in an increase of abdominal fat and glucose intolerance. A study of BPA excretion in urine, sweat, and blood showed the highest levels were detected in sweat from the use of the Thermal Life Sauna.

Far Infrared Sauna Therapy is the most effective way to mobilize BPA from adipose tissue and excrete the toxin through the skin via sweat. Far Infrared detoxification should be a mandatory step to lose weight by removing obesity-causing toxins, while relieving the serious health problems that harm the body when overweight.

Toxicity combined with nutritional deficiency can be very detrimental to your potential to improve your quality of life potential. The body needs nutrients and thrives in a balanced state. When the body is in a toxic overload, it is unable to absorb nutrients. Sauna detoxification will rid the body of destructive toxins that can impede its ability to absorb healthy nutrients. A combination of nutrients and detoxification are essential for restoring and maintaining optimal health.

The human body is smart. Instead of allowing toxins to attack our vital organs, the body protects itself by creating layers of fat cells to store harmful toxins. Far Infrared detoxification increases the body's core temperature to encourage the heavy metals and chemicals to be released from the fat cells and excreted through sweat, breath, urine, and stool. If you want to lose weight, you must detoxify your body of toxins daily. Far Infrared increases metabolism and blood circulation, effectively deals with cellulite, and stimulates the immune system.

High daily stress levels cause constant strain on the body's nervous system and can contribute to chronic disease. Emotional stress is another source of toxins created within the body. Depressive or angry emotions cause the body to release chemicals that weaken our neurological, hormonal, and immune function. Stress places the body at risk for the development of cancer and degenerative diseases. Far Infrared detoxification reduces stress by boosting circulation and triggering the release of endorphins, your feel-good hormones. Far Infrared therapy also relieves the pathways used in the metabolization of stress chemicals, supporting healthy body function.

Solution Provider: The Thermal Life Sauna
by High Tech Health

High Tech Health began advocating Far Infrared Sauna Therapy more than fifteen years ago as an extremely effective way to detoxify the body from heavy metals and chemicals. With the assistance of doctors and engineers, High Tech Health designed the Thermal Life Sauna specifically for detoxification. Today, the Thermal Life Sauna is used by thousands of medical practitioners and their patients worldwide.

The Thermal Life Sauna is made of premium poplar wood, a pure wood that comes from the Aspen family. Unlike cedar, spruce, pine, basswood, and hemlock, poplar is odorless and doesn't emit hydrocarbons that cause lung irritations and contribute to total toxicity.

This type and brand of sauna has state-of-the-art bio-resonance emitters strategically placed throughout the entire cabin, ensuring delivery of the highest quality Far Infrared therapy to the entire body. There is a fresh-air fan in the sauna to keep CO_2 levels low, delivering fresh air to the body and providing the healthiest environment for detoxification.

High Tech Health has certified the Thermal Life Sauna for both home and commercial use to meet and exceed safety requirements for Canada, the United States, and Europe. In order to receive the best results when using infrared saunas, check with High Tech Health for in depth instructions.

For more information on this, visit www.hightechhealth.com. Thermal Life Saunas generally range from $1,000 to $2,000. If you are unable to afford one of these saunas, check around at your local gyms and health spas to see if one is available for you to use.

PRACTICE YOGA TO RELEASE TOXINS

Exercise plays a role in ridding the body of toxins, through perspiration, and yoga has become one of the leading exercise movements in the world. Not only is yoga great exercise but also a powerful stimulant for the entire body and mind; it especially provides a toxin-removing boost, either before or after you use a Far-Infrared sauna.

For insights into the role of yoga, we turned to Angela Grace, a yoga teacher from Boulder, Colorado, who has led yoga retreats and multiple yoga teacher trainings. All opinions and research statements presented in the following paragraphs are from her.

With a laser-focused vision for healing, Angela has overcome personal health challenges, including a debilitating accident, through addressing all aspects of the TDOS Solution, with nutritional fasting, supplements, yoga, and energy medicine.

Angela, with a degree in Mechanical Engineering from the University of Notre Dame, points out how our fascination with science in America can be likened to an obsession. Many times we hear someone state a fact, and a common response might be, "Yes, but is that backed by science?"

What many people don't know is that the first yoga practitioners used scientific principles to develop the practice. They used their own bodies in experiments regarding nutrition, physical exercise, mindfulness techniques, such as meditation, and cleansing practices for the body's systems—cellular, digestive, circulatory, respiratory, and lymphatic. Ayurveda, yoga's sister science, was implemented more than 5,000 years ago.

Ayurveda is an approach to health that considers individual body and psychological constitutions and prescribes practices, such as nutrition, cleansing, massage, yoga postures, and mindfulness practices such as meditation, to heal the body, mind, and spirit.

Yoga was developed and honed based on the anecdotal effectiveness of these techniques and then taught orally from generation to generation, until recently these practices were recorded and, in our modern world, taught mostly through group experiences and sometimes one-on-one in therapeutic settings.

Yoga has become incredibly popular in the US, due largely to the incorporation of this methodology into group classes and the widespread use of video technology to bring yoga instruction into the comfort of people's homes. Students are empowered by being encouraged to listen to their bodies, feel any sensations, and make a shift in their bodies if pain is felt. Having learned this skill, students can transfer it to other parts of their life, such as in their eating practices and stress management.

Imagine wringing out a dirty washcloth, and having whatever dirt is in it come out with the water. Yoga works in much the same way. Various poses create intentional compression in the joints, the abdomen, and the lymph system to detoxify through a wringing effect.

Detoxification is further accomplished through the coordination of the circulatory, digestive, and lymphatic systems. In a healthy body, the circulatory system delivers oxygen to the cells and carries away waste products. When functioning properly, the digestive system processes our food, separates nutrients and waste, transfers nutrients to our bloodstream, and releases waste from the body. The lymphatic system collects intracellular fluids and transports them to the lymph nodes to remove anything harmful before returning it to the bloodstream. Other systems like the glutathione system aid in more robust detoxification.

When our endocrine system is not functioning properly, this sets up a chain reaction, presenting many health challenges. Some yoga poses work to support glands, such as the thyroid, adrenals, and pituitary, to return to a balanced state that corrects deficiencies.

Yoga is different than other forms of exercise because it has a therapeutic effect on all major systems of the body, and it focuses on both stretching and compressing the body, facilitating greater detoxification. Yoga can be very effective with as little as practicing two or three times a week.

BEGIN NUTRITIONAL FASTING
TO LEACH OUT TOXINS

Vibrant health, which requires shedding the body burden of toxins, is greatly dependent on using a new approach that we call nutritional fasting, which allows the body to naturally remove toxins from our systems. This is in no way a traditional fast. It is a revolutionary new nutritional fasting approach, and a core facet of the TDOS Solutions.

Nutritional fasting is based on caloric reduction *but not nutritional reduction*. It relies on nutritional density—by making every calorie count. Therein lies its secret to success. It works by reducing the number of calories consumed, while maintaining a high nutritional density. Although the number of calories is reduced, as in traditional fasting, the difference in *nutritional* fasting is that these calories are loaded with nutrients. Therefore, the body receives all the benefits of fasting without entering into starvation mode. (I will explain nutritional fasting in much greater detail in chapter five.)

The good news about eliminating toxins is that the human body is incredibly resilient. It can naturally rid itself of toxins so they no longer feed the three other deadly co-factors of the TDOS Syndrome—nutrient deficiencies, overweight, and stress.

The problem is that if you rely only on current food choices—and strategies like diet and exercise—to combat toxicity, you will probably be greatly disappointed in their effectiveness. There is a whole host of co-factors to consider: very specific nutrients, vitamins, botanicals, major minerals, essential trace minerals, and trace elements. These co-factors, though invisible (and calorie-less), must be combined to magnify their effectiveness and to create the best offensive strategy against toxicity.

For the purposes of this book, we will refer to the essential major (macro) minerals, essential trace (micro) minerals, and essential trace elements as "the mineral suites." We will walk you through the natural botanicals, vitamins, and mineral suites that will maximize your body's toxin-hunting capabilities. You will also learn how to most effectively consume them to maximize the body's ability to naturally clear out toxins.

What to Take and How to Take It

The first step is choosing the right array of these micronutrients. The second step is following a specific, day-by-day regimen that gives your body the time and resources it needs to naturally rid you of toxins.

Always keep in mind that it is your body doing the detoxifying. The formulas and recipes we provide give your body massive amounts of nutrients in very few calories. But it is our bodies that use these nutrients to fuel their fight against the toxins in our systems. Our bodies are the real miracle here, not the nutritional approach we introduce.

Total detox requires a specific combination of nutrients, including proteins (from either grass-fed dairy cows or from specific vegan formulas) with a high percentage of amino acids, botanicals, and the critically important essential mineral suites.

Why Is Protein So Important?

To have a healthy body, you need to have the right carefully selected proteins every day. The human body stores fats and carbohydrates, but *it does not store protein.* This is why regular consumption of the right protein is a health essential.

In addition to water, protein also comprises a large percentage of our bodies. If one were to drain all the fluids from the body, the remainder would be about half protein. That's right—about half of your dry body weight is protein. In fact, protein, specifically whey protein, may be the single most important nutrient for the human body. It is clearly not just for building muscles. Proteins are in nearly every cell in our body, including our brain. But the right *kind* of protein really matters for maximizing our quality of life potential.

Not All Whey Protein Is Created Equal

Michael Colgan, PhD, is one of the world's leading experts on protein. Along with his research team, he has analyzed nearly every protein source on the planet, including proteins from animals, plants, and even seaweed. He has concluded that carefully selected, raw, undenatured whey protein from grass-fed dairy cows is one of the best protein options in the world.

Carefully selected, raw, undenatured whey proteins can be found in many regions of the world, including Canada, the US, Mexico, England, Switzerland, Italy, Germany, Australia, New Zealand, and many other countries. It doesn't matter where you find them, as long as the carefully selected, raw, undenatured whey proteins meet key considerations (criteria) we discovered through our extensive research as outlined below.

Dr. Colgan has made it clear that after researching proteins for more than 30 years, he has discovered that these incredibly complex substances are not all the same. Some protein sources are much healthier and supply more usable protein than others.

The ideal whey protein has unique properties, some of which mimic mothers' breast milk, humanity's first perfect food. Therefore, carefully selected raw whey protein shakes contain approximately the same protein in amounts almost identical to the same ratios of protein and milk protein found in human breast milk. Comparatively, typical cow's milk that has been pasteurized does not come close to those ratios.

These carefully selected raw whey proteins are excellent sources of all the essential amino acids, but they differ in one important aspect. Whey is a fast-digesting protein, and casein (another milk protein) is a slow-digesting protein. This means milk protein works to keep amino acid levels in the blood steady over a longer period of time and to promote optimal muscle growth.

What to Look for When Selecting Whey Protein

There are several key considerations when selecting your raw whey protein.

First, whey protein should originate from cows that have not been injected with growth hormones or antibiotics or whose food sources are not riddled with herbicides and pesticides. Second, the cows need to be only grass fed not corn or grain fed.

In his book *The Omnivore's Dilemma*, Michael Pollan pointed out that feeding corn or grains to cows destroys their immune system. Cows are ruminants and they were meant to eat grass—not corn or grains. Because a diet of corn or grains weakens their immune system, they must be given anti-biotics or they become sick. Pollan also explained that we eat whatever a plant or animal has ingested, including antibiotics and hormones that are often injected into livestock and poultry. There is a wide belief that this is a major contributor to the scary reality of our growing resistance to antibiotics. We should only get antibiotics or hormones from a prescription—not from what we eat.

Study after study confirms the negative effects on human health from ingesting corn-fed animal proteins. Fortunately, there are more and more sources now for grass-fed, hormone-free, and antibiotic-free animal proteins. We consumers have a lot of power in our wallets. If we create the demand, more and more supermarkets will carry a supply of grass-fed, hormone-free, and antibiotic-free animal proteins. The authors, including Dr. Messina, eat organic, grass-fed, hormone-free, antibiotic-free animal proteins whenever possible.

Third, and most important, the whey should not be denatured; it needs to be undenatured. "Undenatured" means that the processing of whey is not done with high heat pasteurization, as is the norm in North America. High temperature pasteurization breaks the protein folds that contain amino acids. This high heat diminishes the use of the amino acids in the human body. The processing should be a low-temperature, high-filtration process. It is critically important that you source your raw whey protein with the above considerations in mind if you want the best possible results.

Our bodies are composed of more than 20,000 different kinds of proteins, some of them formed in amino acid chains more than 30,000 in length. This means that to be healthy and full of vitality, we need to consume protein sources that provide everything we need. Colgan believes that protein may be the single most important nutrient, and many of us are simply not getting enough of it.

Dr. Colgan also confirms something I've known for years: Cooking meat as a source of protein is not the best option for getting the protein you need. Cooking causes the protein to become denatured, a term referring to the breakdown of natural folds in a protein's structure. In short, any high heat processing of proteins (as used in most pasteurization processes in North American countries) causes them to be denatured, which means the natural protein folds break down.

What are the best sources of raw whey protein powder on planet Earth? Carefully selected, raw, undenatured whey protein powder that has the qualities we mentioned above. It may take a little work on your part to source out the best raw whey proteins. Your body will thank you for the extra effort.

Now that you know what to look for, keep in mind it is what the cows eat and how the whey is processed that become some of the determining factors in your quest for the best raw whey protein sources. It is important that when you source your raw whey protein it includes the specific properties we have laid out in this book. Again, our goal is to make you aware of what should be included on the ingredient list.

Whey Protein Reduces Oxidative Stress

According to an article published by the U.S. National Library of Medicine and the National Institutes of Health,[2] researchers have reason to believe that undenatured whey is better than denatured. The reason for this is because while denatured whey is broken down into individual amino acids, undenatured whey protein is processed in such a way that the protein's "natural folds" are left. The researchers who conducted the study say there's evidence that undenatured whey protein is better able to boost antioxidants and enhance the immune system.

The study further states that oxidative stress occurs when harmful oxidative agents created through psychological, dietary, or environmental stress, or the natural metabolic process, overwhelm our antioxidant systems, damaging cells. Whey protein is an excellent source of the building blocks of glutathione, which is one of the most important antioxidants in terms of protecting cells from injury and slowing the aging process.

As we age, our ability to manufacture glutathione decreases, making whey protein especially important for seniors. In fact, the NLM-NIH study revealed that some people in their 60s and 70s have glutathione levels that are as much as 50 percent lower than those who are in their 20s and 30s. This demonstrates how important whey protein is in fighting oxidative stress and slowing down the cellular aging process.

Glutathione and Selenium Fight Toxins

As mentioned above, glutathione found in whey protein is an important antioxidant It is a critical substance for detoxifying the liver and every cell in the body. Its production depends on the availability of several amino acids, along with available iron and an important trace mineral called selenium. Together these form the enzyme glutathione peroxidase, which is a step in glutathione production and metabolism.

When glutathione production is low, detoxification in the liver is seriously impaired. This means the body is less able to eliminate all toxic metals, many toxic chemicals, and other substances such as biological toxins.

Glutathione is needed in every cell in the body to protect cell membranes, cell proteins, and DNA. It is also one of two primary ways the body detoxifies itself. Most glutathione is produced naturally in the body, but the toxins contained in most foods today diminish glutathione levels.

There are supplements available containing glutathione or glutathione-sparing nutrients. However, these nutrient supplements can be difficult for the body to absorb and may only provide minor benefits. A far better solution would be to take in glutathione in responsibly-sourced whey protein. Carefully selected whey proteins are high in the amino acid cysteine, which has been shown to significantly boost glutathione levels in the body. It is always better for the body to make more glutathione on its own than to take a glutathione supplement.

This is a great example of interconnectivity and the effectiveness of the TDOS Solutions' combination of magnifying forces to combat the "S" and chronic oxidative stress in the TDOS Syndrome.

Additional Important Ingredients

We need to be cognizant of preventive interventional strategies as the best way to maximize our quality of life potential. Approaches such as simply not eating meat from animals that were fed corn or injected with antibiotics or growth hormones are an easy step toward a healthier lifestyle. You may want to consume products from grass-fed cows every chance you get in order to avoid ingesting additional toxins.

Drinking a shake made from carefully selected raw whey protein is a wonderful way to begin to rid your body of toxins. But whey on its own is still not enough. The first thing to look for when selecting a whey protein is to make sure the product label specifies that the protein is undenatured. This specific process of production is a critical piece when selecting a world-class whey protein.

A number of other substances should be included in any carefully selected whey protein you purchase. It is important to read your labels to see if what you are buying contains some if not all of these additional ingredients.

Lactase, Lipase, and Protease Enzymes

Any carefully selected whey protein shake should contain the enzyme lactase. This is to aid anyone who may be lactose intolerant, although carefully selected whey protein contains very low levels of lactose.

Lactose intolerance affects many people. Therefore, to cut down on the likelihood of a negative reaction to protein powders, the ingredient of lactase can allow many who have lactose intolerance to still experience the many health benefits derived from Whey protein powders. Of course, it does not guarantee (as nothing is 100 percent effective) that you might still have a reaction.

So, if you decide to try a whey shake with lactase, take a little bit of the shake and see if you have any side effects before consuming a whole shake.

The Lipase Enzyme

Another very important enzyme to look for on the label is the enzyme Lipase.

Lipase is derived from the Green word "lipos," which is the word for fat.

One of the main functions of lipase is to break down fat in to smaller molecules to make them more digestible so they can pass out of the body. The breakdown of fat also prevents it from coating food particles and thus inhibiting the breakdown of proteins and carbohydrates (that are in the shakes).

People with lipase deficiencies could be more prone to have high triglycerides and high cholesterol. That is because lipase helps to digest fat and fat soluble vitamins.

It should be obvious that a shake without lipase is not going to be as good for the body as having lipase to help extract the necessary components for maximizing our high quality of life potential.

Protease Enzymes

Equally important is the enzyme protease, since protease is specifically needed by the body to break down protein into tiny particles called peptides. This leads to much easier absorption of the amino acids into our cells. By sourcing whey protein from carefully selected sources that can be found around the world and include proteases in particular, you're able to get a higher utilization of the amino acids in this whey protein.

Protease greatly increases what is called the bioavailability of amino acids, the pieces that really matter in protein molecules. This simply means that with the addition of protease, the body will have a much easier time using all the necessary building blocks of life with very little waste from inefficient absorption.

It is important to understand that what really matters is not what we eat or drink, but what we actually absorb. A good analogy is someone with pulmonary issues who has difficulty breathing. He or she might get the same amount of oxygen as the rest of us, but the lung tissue has a hard time absorbing the oxygen in the air. It's the same with the food that we eat: If we lack sufficient protease, we simply don't absorb all of the amino acids that we need, and all those good proteins pass through our bodies unused.

Pre-Biotic Fiber

You may also want to add prebiotic (not probiotic) fiber, also known as Isomaltooligosaccharides, because prebiotic fiber creates good flora (gut bacteria) in the colon. Most people are familiar with probiotic fiber, which is widely advertised. Probiotic fiber is based on the old health conversation of a "defensive procedural intervention"—using probiotics to help with health challenges, such as to remedy heartburn or an upset stomach. Also, far too rarely, doctors suggest that patients take probiotics after taking an antibiotic regimen in order to restore gut flora. But we want to go even further.

It is much better to be on the offense by using prebiotic fiber to avoid gut problems in the first place. This is a key point in the new health conversation. But don't be fooled into thinking that relying on probiotics is the only way to go. It is not. The use of probiotics in addition to prebiotics can be an effective strategy as well. If you can only afford one, we recommend the prebiotic fiber.

It is also critically important that you understand that prebiotic fiber also helps to regulate the release of insulin, thus avoiding insulin spikes. This is a fact that should not be overlooked. It is important to understand that in the end you want a shake with a low glycemic index and a low glycemic load. It is not necessarily the amount of sugar that is used but in fact how it is released into the bloodstream. Many times, people look at labels of shakes and say, "oh there is too much sugar." Instead, they should be more concerned with whether the shake has prebiotic not probiotic fiber to regulate the release of glucose. A good example is found in nature. Eating an orange or an apple is completely different than drinking orange juice or apple juice. Nature made an orange and an apple; it did not make orange juice or apple juice. The fiber is there for a reason: to modulate and regulate the release of the natural sugars contained in an apple, orange, grapefruit, or other fruits. If you are drinking orange juice, at least get it labeled containing pulp or fiber.

What Sweeteners Are Best?

There are several sweeteners that you can use. These range from sugar from sugar beets, honey, black strap molasses, and stevia. We do not recommend the use of artificial sweeteners. Also, keep in mind if you are using a sweetness source, you must use prebiotic fiber for the best effect in your body. The low glycemic index and low glycemic load are very important.

Also, do not be fooled by the labels on meal replacement shakes in stores when they say low sugar and yet they only contain 100 calories. This is totally misleading since the FDA requires that for a shake to be classified as a meal replacement it must contain 240 calories. So, in essence, when you are looking at the label and it says "10 grams of sugar in 100 calories," you would need to consume two-and-a-half shakes to equal the minimum for a meal replacement. In other words, it would now be 25 grams of sugar (10 grams for 100 calories × 2.5 = 25 grams). It is so important that you know what you are looking at when you are trying to formulate or find a source of your carefully selected, raw, undenatured whey protein formulations.

Selenium

Many of the thousands of research studies on glutathione have revealed that un-denatured whey protein is a great way to boost glutathione levels. The research we have seen indicates that the micro mineral (or trace mineral) selenium is a co-factor for cysteine, making it more effective. Cysteine plays a huge part in boosting glutathione levels.

As we have discussed, there is a wide array of minerals that make up the mineral suite profile. The micro-mineral selenium is just one of many that will need to be added to any shake you drink. Specific shake recipes can be found in part II and part III of this book. If you are a vegan, we recommend you consume the vegan shake recipes we outline later.

QUICK REFERENCE FOR OPTIMAL SHAKE INGREDIENTS

24-36 grams of undenatured whey protein free from antibiotics and growth hormones and processed through a low-temperature, high-filtration pasteurization, pre-biotic fiber from flax seed, The enzymes (lipase, lactase, protease), vitamin D-3, oleic acid, the "mineral suites" (essential major (macro) minerals, essential trace (micro) minerals, and essential trace elements), good fats (olive oil, sunflower oil, and coconut oil). Stevia is okay as a sweetener.

Avoid: artificial sweeteners, soy or soy-derived ingredients, GMO ingredients, and make sure shakes are gluten free.

*   *   *

Keep in mind that using any of the TDOS Solutions is about progress, not perfection. The more you do to avoid allowing toxins to enter your body, the better off you are. The more informed you are as to what you put into your body, the more prepared you are to defeat the toxins. You can begin alleviating your body burden by using Far Infrared Saunas as often as possible, regularly practicing yoga, and beginning a program of nutritional fasting that incorporates carefully sourced, raw, undenatured whey proteins, lactase and protease enzymes, pre-biotic fiber, and selenium.

In order to maximize your quality of life potential, it is critical that you integrate these solutions into your lifestyle. None of the solutions or ideas presented in this book are quick fixes. Feel free to pick and choose what works best for you but don't pretend that one detox or one week of yoga will eliminate all the junk in our bodies forever. In the next chapter, we will look more specifically at the types of minerals that need to be added to your diet to overcome the nutritional deficiencies that undermine your body's ability to fight toxins.

Chapter Two

Nutrient Deficiency Interventions

The following is a summary of the problem of nutrient deficiency (as identified in our first book, *The TDOS Syndrome*):

- The "dumbing down" of our food supply, as a result of nutrient depletion in food crops, began with the wholesale introduction of agricultural techniques in the 20th century that relied on chemical engineering (pesticides, herbicides, chemical fertilizers, GMOs, and so on) to increase harvests.

- Food scientists compared the mineral content of 20 fruits and 20 vegetables grown in the 1930s, on through the 1980s, and discovered numerous big reductions in mineral content, particularly in the levels of calcium, magnesium, copper, and sodium in vegetables, and magnesium, iron, copper, and potassium in fruits.

- A 2009 study in the *Journal of HortScience* found, for instance, that fruits and vegetables taste worse today than they did in past generations, and the average vegetable found in grocery stores today has up to 40 percent fewer minerals than the average from 50 years ago.

- Nutrient depletion has been further accelerated by processing practices used in the creation of convenience foods and fast foods, and by cooking methods that fried, boiled, baked, and steamed remaining nutrients from the foods.

- Eating organic fruits and vegetables lowers exposure to pesticides, but organic foods offer few advantages over non-organic when it comes to mineral and vitamin content, especially in providing some of the mineral elements from the soil (such as copper, magnesium, and zinc) that have been identified as essential to human health.

- "Nutrient deficiencies occur {even in populations eating} a balanced and varied diet," observed a 2014 study in *Nutrition Journal*, "including in populations with bountiful food supplies and the means to procure nutrient-rich foods. For example, the typical American diet bears little resemblance to what experts recommend for fruit, vegetables, and whole grains. With time, deficiencies in one or more micronutrients may lead to serious health issues."

- Nutrient deficiencies start in the womb, before birth. It is well accepted in medical circles that a pregnant woman, deficient in nutrients, can contribute to stunting the growth and development of an unborn child. As these children grow and become adults, they are more susceptible to becoming overweight, as well as suffering from chronic diseases, including diabetes and hypertension.

- Nutrient deficiencies, along with toxins, are directly connected to becoming overweight. We over-eat empty calories filled with salt, sugar, and fat. There is no substance in these calories to satisfy the body's need for nutrition. Without nutritionally dense foods, hunger intensifies, and so does weight gain.

MINERAL SUITES: THE SPARK PLUGS OF LIFE

Can a car run without spark plugs? Can a body run without what we call the "mineral suites"? The answer to both of these questions should be a resounding NO. Many people are unfamiliar with the critically important role that these mineral suites play in the optimal functioning of the human body. Even worse, many of these life-supporting minerals have almost vanished from our earthly foods. There are approximately 60 or more chemical elements found in varying amounts in the human body. In order to save time, we coined the term "Mineral Suites." The mineral suites will always include: Essential Major (Macro Minerals), Essential Trace (Micro Minerals), Essential Trace Elements, and Nonessential Trace Elements still considered to be beneficial.

Twenty of those chemical elements are comprised of essential major minerals, essential trace minerals, and essential trace elements that are needed by the human body. There are an additional 6 trace elements, found to be beneficial but not essential to human health.

ESSENTIAL MINERALS THAT THE BODY NEEDS

What we call the "mineral suites" are the essential minerals that are sometimes divided up into the categories of major minerals (macro minerals), trace minerals (micro minerals) and trace elements. These three groups of minerals are equally important, but trace minerals and trace elements are needed in smaller amounts than major minerals. The amounts needed in the body are not an indication of their importance since they are all integral for proper body function. A balanced, healthy diet needs to provide all of the following essential minerals.

Essential Major (Macro) Minerals:

- Sodium
- Chloride

- Potassium
- Calcium
- Phosphorus
- Magnesium
- Sulfur

Essential Trace (Micro) Minerals:

- Iron
- Zinc
- Iodine
- Selenium
- Copper
- Manganese
- Fluoride
- Chromium
- Molybdenum

Essential Trace Elements:

- Silicon
- Vanadium
- Cobalt
- Nickel

Nonessential Trace Elements Considered to be Beneficial:

- Bromine
- Lithium
- Strontium
- Silicon
- Vanadium
- Cadmium

The severe depletion of these major minerals, trace minerals, and trace elements from the soil—and thus from our food—is one of the most significant parts of co-factor "D" (nutritional deficiency) in the TDOS Syndrome. The mineral suites make up a huge part of the periodic table and are the most significant nutrients missing from our food today, even if that food is organic and even if it is home-grown. They include minerals such as potassium, magnesium, iron, zinc, selenium, boron, nickel, and others.

Before I began implementing the TDOS Solutions in my own life, these important elements from the mineral suites were either missing from my daily food intake entirely, or they were present in amounts that weren't high enough to make a difference. It wasn't until I started using nutrient-dense calories (containing all the necessary nutrients, vitamins, botanicals, and the full spectrum of the mineral suites) that were being formulated in new nutritional approaches that my own health began to rapidly improve.

From the first moment that I consumed massive amounts of nutrients, vitamins, and the mineral suites to replenish these miss-ing nutrients in my body, my frequent food cravings for sugar and simple carbohydrates disappeared. It was only when I started using this approach of caloric reduction and nutritional fasting that my body received appropriate life-changing elements.

More than 35 years ago, a US patent was awarded for the extraction of these minerals for human consumption from ancient plant deposits that were millions of years old. It has only been in the last ten years that the use of all these elements existing in ancient mineral suites in our Earth were formulated as new nutritional approaches that cen-tered on the new concept of nutritional density. These nutritionally dense ingredients treat the body as a whole, supplying it with massive amounts of nutrients, vitamins, and the all-so-critical mineral suites. Now, my body performs the way it was designed and self-regulates to achieve optimal health.

It is possible to re-mineralize the soil. In other words, to put the minerals back in the soil is possible today, but the expense is enormous. So, what can we do? The solution is to obtain mineral supplement support that contains the macro minerals, micro minerals, and essential as well as nonessential trace elements. The formulas that we reveal to you in this book are based on your supplementing your food sources with these mineral suites.

Even medical doctors are sometimes unaware of the significance of these combined minerals and trace elements. Regarding our health, Nicholas Messina, MD, stated, "While conducting research for the TDOS Syndrome and Solutions, it occurred to me how little time was spent during my medical education on nutrition. As I look back over my medical career, I can't help but wonder how recommending the consumption of the mineral suites and 16 vitamins, 12 amino acids, and three essential fatty acids required daily for optimum health and longevity could have altered the outcomes for many of my patients."

Let's begin by taking a close look at the significance of these minerals and trace elements to our wellness potential, and why the loss of them can be so devastating.

It is nearly impossible to overestimate the importance of the balance of the different categories of minerals in maintaining and supporting our overall health. In fact, it's been noted that "Although minerals comprise only a fraction of total body weight (less than 4 percent), they are crucial for many bodily functions including transporting oxygen, normalizing the nervous system, simulating growth, and maintenance and repair of tissues and bones."[3] That's right—although minerals make up only about 4 percent of total body weight, they are absolutely essential to allowing our bodies to function at or near our maximum quality of life potential.

MAJOR MINERALS OR MACRO MINERALS

Minerals are essential for the production of vitamins, enzymes, and hormones in the body as well as for proper blood circulation, fluid regulation, nerve transmission, muscle contraction, cellular integrity and energy production. These minerals work synergistically with each other and with other nutrients. Macro minerals are present at larger levels in the human body and are required in larger amounts in the diet. The major minerals of the human body in this mineral suite traditionally include the following, as shown on the periodic table:

- Calcium
- Phosphorus
- Magnesium
- Sodium
- Potassium
- Chloride
- Sulfur

MICRO MINERALS OR TRACE MINERALS

A precise definition for the essential micro minerals (or trace minerals or trace elements) has not been established. These minerals initially gained their description "trace" because their concentrations in tissue were not easily quantified by early analytical methods. Today, however, trace minerals can be analyzed by a variety of techniques. The term "trace," when applied to minerals or elements, is still used and can be defined as minerals that make up less than 0.01 percent of total body weight.

The category of this mineral suite includes the following nine essential micro minerals (or trace minerals):

- Iron
- Zinc

- Copper
- Iodine
- Selenium
- Molybdenum
- Manganese
- Chromium
- Fluoride

Recommended dietary allowances (RDA) have been established for humans for these essential trace minerals. Adequate intakes have been estimated for another three trace minerals (fluoride, manganese, and chromium).

Each essential micro mineral is necessary for one or more functions in the body. Each mineral's function(s), like those of other essential nutrients, are optimal when mineral intake and body concentrations of the nutrient fall within a specific range. These biochemical changes can be prevented or cured when the deficiency is prevented or cured.

Others define trace elements as nutrients the body needs in concentrations of one part per million or less. An element is considered essential if a dietary deficiency of that element consistently results in a subsequent biological function that is preventable or reversible by physiological amounts of the element.

TRACE ELEMENTS

Trace elements have been defined as those mineral elements with estimated, established, or suspected requirements of less than 1 mg/day. Based on this definition, as many as 13 elements may be classified in our "mineral suite" as trace elements. They include:

- Aluminum
- Boron

- Bromine
- Cadmium
- Chromium
- Copper
- Germanium
- Lithium
- Molybdenum
- Nickel
- Rubidium
- Silicon
- Vanadium

WHAT DO TRACE MINERAL ELEMENTS DO FOR OUR BODIES?

Even in minute portions, minerals can powerfully affect health. These "mineral suites" are necessary for oxygen transport, energy metabolism, growth, and cell and nerve protection. The combined impacts of the right combinations of the mineral categories are essential for the assimilation and utilization of vitamins and other nutrients. They aid in the digestion process and provide the catalyst for many hormones, enzymes, essential body functions, and reactions. They aid in replacing electrolytes lost through heavy perspiration, or diarrhea, and also protect against toxic reaction and heavy metal poisoning.

The body can use essential minerals and elements without vitamins, but vitamins and most other nutrients are basically useless in the absence of minerals and elements, no matter how small the requirement may be. Research has also proven that without adequate nutrients, including essential major minerals and trace minerals and trace elements, our cells experience a breakdown that can lead to chronic conditions.

The body must be supplied with proper nutrients, botanicals, vitamins, essential minerals, and trace elements to optimally function. We can certainly use the necessary support of the essential minerals and trace elements to speed up detoxification and antioxidant enzyme reactions in the body. The micro mineral selenium is needed to produce glutathione peroxidase, which in turn combats oxidative stress. Zinc is essential for many enzymes, and cobalt is part of vitamin B_{12}, as well as the vehicle to efficiently open cells to receive and process nutrients.

The mineral suites support the majority of muscle functionality in the human body and the key components of most body processes. While the essential minerals and trace elements are performing so many functions, they also help eliminate our cravings for sugar and carbohydrates.

We are particularly concerned with plant-based essential micro minerals (or trace minerals), because they are have almost completely vanished from our soils and thus from our food supply.

Our research on minerals leads us to a major conclusion: that essential minerals are one of if not *the* most important co-factors of the TDOS Solution's multifaceted approach to attack and eliminate the TDOS Syndrome. Any strategy to effectively fight the negative and destructive force of the TDOS Syndrome should include essential minerals and essential trace elements.

Arden Andersen, MD, has effectively demonstrated that, "in order to change human health, we have to go back and change the soil, because that's where it comes from. And that's really where preventive medicine begins—right in the soil."[4]

However, the necessary change to farming practices and hence, to our soil, is unlikely to happen any time soon. This means that food alone is simply not enough to supply us with the minerals that our bodies need to be healthy. **Even following a clean, organic diet with plenty of vegetables, the average number of minerals found is roughly ten.**

Extensive research shows that without supplementation, it is nearly impossible to eat enough food to obtain the full range of essential minerals and trace elements required to obtain optimum health and longevity. For those who think you are doing everything right from a nutritional standpoint, you might be shocked to know that food will never be enough again. Unless you are ingesting botanicals, vitamins, sufficient nutrients, and a broad array of the essential minerals from the mineral suites, you are robbing your body of its maximum wellness potential. It is simply naïve to think that we can get the vitamins, nutrients and minerals, and trace elements from our food alone; all evidence suggests that we cannot.

We must then supplement our diet with other mineral sources. Basically, we have two options for mineral supplements: colloidal minerals and ionic minerals. And ionic major minerals and micro minerals are by far the better choice. It can be quite difficult to track down the 26 major minerals, trace minerals, and trace elements that have been shown to benefit the body even in health food stores. If you do find them, they are often split among different supplements and are generally expensive. Online, there are a handful of supplement fulfillment companies that offer products that meet these standards.

COLLOIDAL MINERALS VERSUS IONIC MINERALS

According to Chris Meletis, ND, many manufacturers claim that colloidal minerals are in a natural form and therefore are more easily absorbed by the body. However, as Dr. Meletis points out, there is simply "no scientific evidence to support these claims." Instead, Dr. Meletis recommends ionic minerals, which are much easier for the body to efficiently absorb. Ionic minerals contain an electrical charge at the molecular level, which means that the body can easily break them down and absorb them through cell walls.

The good news is that we have an effective recipe for combating nutritional deficiency and turning it into nutritional abundance. Simply by finding fulfillment companies that will either supply a super whey or super vegan shake, whey protein snacks, the inner heart aloe vera with added minerals, specific vitamins, and cleansing botanicals all described later, you will supply the body with huge amounts of nutrients. Your body has been deprived of these massive amounts of nutrients and will function more optimally once they are replenished.

If you only follow *TDOS Solutions'* new nutritional approaches and ignore the rest of *TDOS Solutions* many other co-factors, you will achieve a large part of the solution to nutritional deficiency.

There is still more that we can do to ensure that we are maximizing our quality of life potential by giving our bodies what they require. We can further promote nutritional abundance by ingesting inner heart gel from the aloe vera plant, eating raw foods, consuming sprouts, and eating organic whenever possible.

INNER HEART GEL FROM THE *ALOE* PLANT

You can further support your health with an Aloe vera made from the inner heart filet of aloe vera leaves that have been processed at low temperatures and spray dried to preserve the enzymes and nutrients. The gel is where the leaf stores the majority of its nutrients, enzymes, essential amino acids, vitamins, and minerals, which support digestive health and the immune system while encouraging detoxification.

Also, the inner filet contains special polysaccharides that have been studied for their ability to balance the immune system, and their actions as natural detoxifiers (what we call Toxin Hunters) help move along biochemical processes in the liver to neutralize toxins. Many other Aloe vera supplements crush the leaf and the whole plant. The problem with this type of processing that includes the whole leaf is that the leaf contains an enzyme that actually destroys the polysaccharides and other nutrients. So, the type of Aloe vera you consume really does matter.

In addition to the beneficial effects of utilizing only the inner heart filet of Aloe vera that includes some essential major minerals, micro minerals, and trace elements), the Aloe vera product should also include bilberries, blueberries, and raspberries—all of which serve as great sources of antioxidants and are designed to work with all other nutrients to advance the nutritional fasting processes. Look for an Aloe vera product that includes all these in a powder or liquid form.

QUICK REFERENCE FOR
OPTIMAL DETOX DRINK INGREDIENTS

Aloe vera gel made from the inner heart filet of the *Aloe* plant. Whole leaf aloe cannot be used. Gel must also be processed using a low temperature, spray dry technique in order to preserve the enzymes and nutrients. Aloe vera gel also includes polysaccharides (the natural Toxin Hunters) and to ensure optimization, the detox drink should also include essential and nonessential minerals from the Mineral Suites as well as bilberries, blueberries, and raspberries.

EATING RAW BOOSTS NUTRITIONAL ABUNDANCE

Once you understand that vegetables are already terribly nutritionally deficient, why would you want to further contribute to nutritional deficiency by cooking, boiling, steaming, or, worse yet, microwaving your vegetables? The temperature at which you begin to destroy the enzymes and nutrients is a wet temperature of 118 degrees Fahrenheit and a dry heat temperature of 150 degrees Fahrenheit.

There are many good reasons to eat raw. In his article "10 Reasons Eating Raw is Healthier for You and the Planet,"[5] Jonathan Mead shares his experiences with eating 100 percent raw foods. Some of the benefits or eating raw include preserving and ultimately ingesting more enzymes. The minute that food is cooked over flame or heated, in most cases this method of preparing food kills of most of the beneficial enzymes in our foods. People often notice benefits from sleeping better to a heightened sense of mental clarity. Also, the increase of fiber from a raw diet usually leads to an improved regularity of bowel movements, which leads to better health. The reasons to eat raw are compelling, but, as always, the choice is yours.

SPROUTS ARE NUTRITIONAL POWERHOUSES

In addition to eating raw whenever possible, consuming sprouts can contribute to nutritional abundance. When my coauthors and I first started to write this book, I knew nothing about sprouts. Fortunately, I have been taught a great deal about sprouts by a friend of mine, Michelle Lauber who has researched and used sprouts in her every-day life. Michelle and her husband, prominent anesthesiologist Bernd Lauber, MD, are living the TDOS Solutions to the fullest.

Since becoming aware of the solution and the new nutritional approaches available to them, the Lauber's buy proteins from grass-fed animals, only use organic eggs, and consume most vegetables raw. They also grow and regularly consume sprouts. The Laubers have seen amazing changes in their lives and the lives of their children.

Sprouts are easy and inexpensive to grow. They require little to no maintenance. Sprouts grow from seeds in only four to ten days and need almost no light. I have come to realize that sprouts are an amazing and affordable gift we can all give ourselves. Although little known, sprouts can greatly increase nutritional abundance and at the same time greatly improve your offensive approach to prevention. The miracle of sprouts is that they contain very large quantities of nutrients in a very small package.

We cannot thank Michelle Lauber enough for writing about the amazing properties of sprouts for our book[*] and explaining why you will want to include them in your preventative, interventional diets.

---

[*] The article "*The Amazing Benefits of Sprouts*" is provided by Michelle Lauber. All rights reserved.

According to Michelle, sprouting was popular in the 1970s but lost its fame when the green revolution began punching out cheap, low nutritious foods.

The Amazing Benefits of Sprouts

Now sprouting is experiencing a comeback and it couldn't come at a better time!

Sprouting is the fun, easy, inexpensive, and nutritious way of growing your own food, right in your own kitchen. From seed to feed in about four to ten days, depending on the seeds grown, you can literally produce for yourself and your family a variety of fresh, intensively healthy, deliciously edible food. Sprouts are considered one of the ultimate raw super foods. They are filled with incredible amounts of vitamins, micronutrients, trace minerals, and chemicals to assist the body in combating cancer, asthma, arthritis, and even in helping the body in its detoxification process.

The miracle of these little powerhouses of nutrition is simple to understand once the germination process is explained. A seed is a tremendous storage facility of dormant nutritional energy and vitality. It sits patiently waiting until the right environmental conditions present, such as water and warmth. During the germination process, the seed begins to sprout and natural chemical changes begin to occur. The dormant compounds within the seed undergo a complex biochemical process. As a result, enzymes convert nutrients into smaller compounds in order for the growing plant to utilize them in its own growth process. As this continues, carbohydrates are changed by enzymes into simple sugars. Complex proteins are changed into simple amino acids while fats are converted into fatty acids. All of these new smaller compounds are easier for us to digest.

Vitamins that were once in trace amounts within the seed are now produced in larger quantities during sprouting. For instance, there is very little vitamin C in lentil seeds, but once sprouting occurs, this same vitamin C is increased to the point that it is considered to be a good source in lentil sprouts. The same applies for many different types of sprouts.

There is no other food that provides the same quality of nutritional value in one small serving than sprouts. One of the most healthful benefits of eating sprouts is that they are grown without the use of pesticides and other harmful chemicals. This means they are completely organic in nature. Today, as we've discussed, our food is filled with toxins that overburden the body. The opposite occurs with sprouting. There are no harmful residues of pesticides and herbicides. Sprouting also aids the body in detoxifying by providing the right nutrients that assist the body in this process.

Parents feel safe giving sprouts to their children. Sprouting is an easy, fun way to grow your own food, and kids especially find it fun to grow them.

Watching little seeds turn into healthy, vibrant tiny plants is not only fascinating but also entertaining. Nothing could be more rewarding and educational for children than growing their own food that the entire family can enjoy. All that is needed are several inexpensive materials, such as a mason jar, a 4 × 4 piece of netting (a cut up vegetable wash bag will do), fresh water and seeds. The time commitment is equally as easy. All you need to grow sprouts is an extra minute a day, (30 seconds in the morning and 30 seconds in the evening) for each jar of sprouts you choose to grow.

Most people believe they cannot grow sprouts at home because they do not have enough sunlight to do so. Sprouts, in fact, do not need sunlight to grow. It is yet another one of the miracles of how plants grow. For the first two weeks or so, seeds that are used to sprout have all the energy they need in order to grow. In fact, it's up to the grower whether they want to green up their sprouts in the very last day or so of sprouting. Placing a mason jar of sprouts in a window sill will suffice during the last 24 hours to turn sprouts green, providing more chlorophyll to the plant.

Sprouts are wonderful on salads, sandwiches, and on soups, adding a healthy crunch and fresh flavor to any one of these many meals. A paper created by the International Sprout Grower's Association provided significant research on the health benefits of sprouting. For instance, they found eating sprouts may improve cardiovascular health, and bone mineral density.

Sprouts have the highest concentrations of phytonutrients per calorie than any other food, according to a study by the *International Journal of Applied Science*. Phytonutrients are chemical compounds that naturally occur in plants and have been shown to potentially reduce the risk of cancer. Another significant chemical that has been shown to reduce the risk of cancer is called sulforaphane.

Sulforaphane has been identified in many different sprouts, however in broccoli sprouts they are especially abundant. In fact, broccoli sprouts can have 50–100 times the amount of sulforaphane in a single one-ounce serving than in one-and-a-half cups of broccoli crowns. Sulforaphane not only exhibits anticancer properties but also is known to be antimicrobial.

There is a fairly impressive list of seeds that can be sprouted easily and affordably. One of the best resources on the web for sprouting is www.sproutpeople.org. They not only sell all the materials needed for sprouting but also have detailed videos on the sprouting process. Throughout their website they exhibit the theme that sprouting should be fun and easy, and maybe even a little quirky.

Here is a partial list of seeds that can be used for sprouting:

- Alfalfa
- Broccoli
- Cabbage
- Chia
- Chickpea
- Clover
- Fenugreek
- Leek
- Lentil
- Mung Bean
- Mustard
- Onion
- Pea
- Radish
- Soybean
- Turnip
- Watercress

The list goes on and on. There are a plethora of books, articles, and websites that one can use to become a master sprouter in no time. There are just a few important things to remember when beginning and maintaining a sprouting program:

- Don't be afraid to experiment (after watching a few online videos)
- Have fun watching your sprouts grow!
- When they're all done growing, enjoy the seeds (or vegetables rather than fruits) of your labor, quite literally!
- Share with others about the many benefits of growing sprouts. For, it is in giving that we receive.

Happy Sprouting!!!

CALORIES: QUALITY NOT QUANTITY

A study published in the *Journal of the Medical Association* compared three different eating patterns: a low-fat diet, a low-glycemic-index diet, and a low-carbohydrate diet. The findings illustrated that all calories are not alike from a metabolic perspective. When any major nutrient was avoided or restricted, there was a metabolic consequence noted.

The results suggested it is better to focus not on the quantity of calories, but rather on the quality of nutrients in the calories. This again illustrates that dieting is not enough; food alone will never again be enough. We need better nutrients in our diets.[6]

In addition to carefully selected raw undenatured whey protein shakes and the special Aloe vera drink, you should attempt to eat from the following list of foods. We will also include full recipes as well as the protocols for Nutritional Fasting in chapter eight. (Choose one serving from each column for other meals as a guideline.)

DRINKING HIGH PH WATER:
A NEW NUTRITIONAL APPROACH

Your body, as a whole, is comprised of 60 percent water. The brain alone is 70 to 75 percent water, and your blood is 70 to 83 percent water. Even after consuming a wealth of vitamins, minerals, and nutrients, most people are still deficient in the simplest and most abundant nutrient on Earth: water.

Can drinking alkaline water—or water with a high pH—help? It's still too early to tell, as there have been no definitive peer-reviewed studies, but we believe that drinking water with a high pH has multiple benefits. Essentially, pH measures the level of acidity in your body from 0 – 14, with 1 being highly acidic and 14 being alkaline. Regular water has a pH close to 7, but alkaline waters have a higher pH, ranging from 7 to 9.5.

PROTEIN	GOOD FATS	Fiber-based CARBS
Salmon	Avocado	Romaine Lettuce
Whey Protein (Un-denatured)	Pine Nuts (Raw)	Bell Peppers (All)
Crab/Oysters	Flax Seeds	Green Beans
Tuna	Almonds (Raw)	Celery
Shrimp/Lobster	Walnuts (Raw)	Snow Peas
Halibut	Pecans (Raw)	Zucchini
Canned Sardines	Brazil Nuts (Raw)	Cabbage
Chicken Breast	Tahini	Cucumbers
Lean Beef (95% Fat Free, Grass-Fed and Hormone Free)	Macadamia (Raw)	Broccoli
White Turkey	Avocado Oil (Extra Virgin Cold Pressed)	Artichoke Hearts
Ground Turkey (99% Fat Free)	Almond Butter (Raw Organic)	Asparagus
Rainbow Trout	Coconut Oil Extra Virgin Unrefined Organic)	Cauliflower
Scallops	Almond Oil (Extra Virgin Unrefined Organic)	Endive
Omega 3 Eggs	Raw Butter	Bok Choy

Shannon Brown, CEO of pHenomenal Water, spoke to us about what he feels are the extraordinary benefits of a high pH water, including boundless energy, ridding your body of toxins, a more youthful appearance, and a supercharged immune system that can better fight germs, bacteria and viruses.

According to Brown, "We are surrounded by things that cause our bodies to be in an acidic state—the energy from our hand-held electronic devices, the food we eat, the coffee we drink, the air we breathe, and even the stress we feel when we pay our bills every month. More and more doctors recognize an acidic body is hospitable to disease. Maintaining a proper acid/alkaline balance in your body is the key to unlocking your body's healthiest potential.

But the problem of getting and maintaining a proper balance is a challenge while eating today's diet, breathing today's air, and living in today's stressful, modern world. Since acid nurtures the environment that viruses, bacteria and diseases thrive in, if you can get that acid that wreaks havoc on your health out of your system, guess what happens? You create an inner alkaline environment. And when you are in the alkaline state your body was intended to thrive in, guess what the awesome side effects are? An alkaline body thrives with energy, staves off illness and disease, has clearer thinking, and some say even glows with vibrancy." So how do you best support the body's pH. regulating mechanism to be more alkaline and less acidic? Well, one helpful way is by drinking more water that has a high pH.

There are a number of ways to obtain high alkaline water, including special filters and faucet attachments as well as through bottled waters that have a higher ph. Certain brands, such as Essentia, Iceland Spring, or Enamors tout their high pH levels. You can simply check their labels to find the pH or visit their websites. We feel one of if not the best PH water additive on the market is from pHenomenal Water. For more information on benefits and how to purchase, go to www. pHenomenal.com. Ultimately, while more research clearly needs to be done, we believe that regularly consuming water that has a higher pH and thus lowering the acidity in your body can have a positive impact on the TDOS Syndrome.

*   *   *

MAXIMIZING YOUR QUALITY OF LIFE POTENTIAL FORMULA

The elements of the mineral suites are critical to countering the nutrient depletion in your body, and it's important to consume the proper quantities of essential major minerals, micro (trace) minerals, and trace elements. In addition to supplements, eating raw, ingesting the inner heart gel from the Aloe vera plant, adding sprouts to your diet, and drinking water with a high pH level can all help counteract the TDOS Syndrome. In the next chapter, we'll delve a bit deeper into nutritional fasting as an intervention for overweight as well as alternative solutions such as yoga.

Chapter Three

Overweight Interventions

The following is a summary of the problem of being overweight (as identified in *The TDOS Syndrome*):

- Nearly 500 researchers from 50 countries compared health data from 1990 through 2010 for the Global Burden of Disease report, revealing what they call a massive shift in global health trends.

    Obesity is a worldwide problem, with the US and China having the highest obesity statistics. From 1975 to 2014, global obesity in men tripled, and obesity in women more than doubled. There are now more obese people on the planet than underweight people.

- As waistlines, have ballooned, so have the numbers of diabetes cases directly attributable to this excess weight: Nearly 10 percent of the world's population now has been diagnosed with either type 1 or type 2 diabetes.

- A new scientific discovery has been made about why people become fat: They have been exposed to "obesogens," environmental toxic chemicals that are endocrine (hormone) disrupters.

Obesogens

- Obesogens promote the creation of excess body fat "by altering programming of fat-cell development, increasing energy storage in fat tissue, and interfering with neuroendocrine control of appetite," one study reported.

- These toxic obesogens migrate from mother to fetus, as the fetus develops in the womb, programming the children to unnaturally develop excess fat deposits after being born. As a result, many children are being born to become fat, no matter how much they exercise, or how healthy they eat.

- Among obesogens so far identified: artificial hormones fed to livestock, which become our food sources; plastic pollutants in some food packaging; chemicals added to processed foods; pesticides sprayed on our produce; a marine and agricultural fungicide called tributyltin; phthalates; DDE (a virtually indestructible residue of DDT); and the list goes on.

- The presence of these obesogens helps to explain why up to 87 percent of people who achieve significant weight loss regain the weight within a few years. Excess toxins in the body may be more of an enemy than excess calories.

- Excessive weight in women has become the second largest cause of preventable death in the United States, following only tobacco-related illnesses. Breast cancer may be linked to weight issues in some women, while diabetes and cardiovascular disease afflict others who become overweight or obese.

- Overweight children are much more likely to become obese when they reach adulthood, and they are also much more likely than other children to suffer from cardiovascular diseases, or diabetes, at younger ages. The result is a greater likelihood of disability, or premature death.

• Following a low-calorie, nutrient poor diet places stress on the body, leading to weight gain—completely opposite of the desired outcome Because of toxins and nutrient deficiencies, low-calorie diets stress the body. By lowering the calories, you are also drastically decreasing the nutritional density of the calories you do consume. The body becomes stressed, trying to allocate these nutritionally bankrupt calories to meet all of its needs. The body then acts in response to stress, from all sources, by increasing production of the stress hormone cortisol, which means that by cutting calories, you inadvertently increase your cortisol levels.

• The TDOS Syndrome is one of the primary causes of gaining weight. The four co-factors of TDOS combine and magnify its effects through a process called *interconnectivity*. This combined force is the reason we are losing the battle of the bulge, resulting in weight gain.

NUTRITIONAL FASTING FOR WEIGHT LOSS

As you may recall from our book *The TDOS Syndrome*, I was introduced to a revolutionary new nutritional approach that changed my life.

To my astonishment, in a matter of weeks, I went from a size 42-inch waist to a 34-inch waist, which I have maintained for the past nine years. In all, I lost more than 30 pounds quickly and safely. And, even more important, I continue to be free of the need for prescription drugs, which is a major triumph.

My weight-loss journey began with a system of nutritional fasting, which I describe in detail throughout part II of this book. Here is an overview of the routine:

I started my nutritional fast with a round of two days of a carefully selected whey protein shake, a healthy lunch (600 calories from lean protein and vegetables and salad), an evening meal of whey protein.

Then, the next two days were nutritional fasting days. I followed up the two nutritional fasting days with five days of replacing my breakfast and dinner with carefully selected, raw, undenatured, whey protein shakes for replenishment. This is done so that the body can rest and prepare for another round of serious deep nutritional fasting days. During the replenish days, I also enjoyed a healthy lunch, which included a protein, (my preference was a chicken breast or a piece of fish) and a sizable portion of green vegetables. The carefully selected whey protein shakes provided the perfect combinations of carbohydrates, fats, proteins, major minerals, trace (micro) minerals, and trace elements to continue the fat-burning and nutritional-fasting processes. Throughout the entire nutritional fast, I also included a combination of super vitamins and whey protein snacks to help curb hunger and stimulate my metabolism.

By the time I was a little over a week into the nutritional fast, I was amazed at how many pounds and inches I released as well as the amount of energy I had. I was also drinking half or nearly half of my body weight in ounces of water every day. I quickly realized there was no way this weight loss was just reduced "water weight" because I had significantly increased my water consumption, well past my normal day's intake.

After completing my series of replenish days (between five and seven days based on your discretion), I returned to the two-deep nutritional fasting days and my body resumed intense fat burning. In my experience, these days are great opportunities for the body to really "clean house," naturally removing the remaining toxins, to achieve optimal health and weight loss. Preferably, the deep nutritional fasting is done in two day increments.

Super Shake Feast Days

After completing my second round of deep nutritional fasting days, I was so happy with my results and how great I felt, I chose to continue with an additional five to seven days of carefully selected whey protein super shake "feast days". When we refer to super shake feast days, you have a shake for breakfast, a 400 to 600 calorie meal for lunch, and another 400 to 600 calorie meal for dinner and a shake for dessert. The meals should include a lean healthy protein as well as your choice of vegetables, the greener the better. The protein source should fit in the palm of your hand as a guide to how much to consume.

I continued on this schedule of rotating between the two deep nutritional fasting days followed by a series of replenish days until I was satisfied with my overall health and weight.

For those of you who want to lose more weight, simply continue with an easy program of five to seven or even ten days of super shake feast days, followed by two days of deep nutritional fasting. Repeat this until your desired individual goals are met.

For a list of complete schedules as well as tips and tricks to maximize your nutritional fast, visit our website, www.PeterGreenlaw.com and click on the "Nutritional Cleansing Schedules and Protocols" tab.

HOW DETOXIFICATION AND WEIGHT LOSS OCCUR

While I was on the nutritional fasting solution, I consumed the raw, carefully selected, undenatured whey protein shakes and chewable whey protein wafer supplements that are packed with the same whey protein that is in carefully selected shakes. These wafers helped curb my hunger by providing small amounts of proteins, fats, carbohydrates, and minerals throughout the day. This kept my body in balance and prevented an afternoon crash of energy.

These wafers helped to maintain an overall nutritional balance in my body. The proteins supported lean muscle development, while the carbohydrates broke down into glucose, keeping my brain sharp. These nutritionally dense mini-meals contain organic coconut oil, which is needed to slow down the release of glucose, maintain the body's fat-burning processes, and stimulate metabolism firings (speeds up metabolism and fat burning). It is also ideal to take a mineral supplement that contains the essential mineral suites to give the body additional nutritional fire power.

The last component in the nutritional fasting approach (and formula) is what I like to refer to a combination vitamin and botanical combinations, that assists the body in burning fat without stimulants. These combinations naturally invigorate the body to maintain energy throughout the day while on the nutritional fast. The additional of mineral supplements containing the essential mineral combinations. The vitamin and botanical supplementation should include a variety of natural ingredients, including apple cider vinegar, green tea leaf extract, niacin, cinnamon-dried bark, and cayenne pepper. If you cannot find all of these in one super vitamin, then you can use multiple capsules if necessary to include these recommended ingredients.

These natural nutrients ensure that the body is constantly satisfied with pure nourishment, even on a low-calorie diet. (Keep in mind that these ingredients are for appetite support, and not for appetite suppression.)

WHAT I CONSUMED ON
NUTRITIONAL FASTING DAYS

During my first deep nutritional fasting day, I was only ingesting liquid nutrition in the Aloe vera mineral drink, whey protein wafers, the vitamin and botanicals (listed above) while drinking half my body weight in ounces of water. It surprised me that my body was fed and satisfied with massive amounts of this liquid nutrition. This occurred because my body had all the necessary nutrients and trace minerals, even though my caloric intake was severely reduced. I was pleasantly surprised that I was not hungry. I was in the wonderful world of nutritional abundance, which has nothing to do with calories. The body only cares about nutrients that can be absorbed.

As my body was optimally supplied with the necessary nutrients in minimal calories, it naturally began to cleanse itself by utilizing the massive amounts of these nutrients. I call some of these specific nutrients *toxin hunters*. The job of a toxin hunter is to break down toxins so they become water soluble and pass out harmlessly through the liver and the kidneys. This is also an effective way to reduce the buildup of obesogens, which we are learning is the buildup of synthetic products and toxins that the body did not know how to combat aside from wrapping them in fat cells. When the body receives what, it needs, these obesogens are removed through the same process; they are broken down to become water soluble so they can also exit the body safely and naturally through the liver and kidneys.

The essential mineral suites support enzymes that naturally occur in the body. Impurities stored in fat cells traveled to my liver to be detoxified. The liver then released these impurities as bile or converted them into water-soluble waste to be processed by my liver and excreted from my body through the colon. This process differs from a colon cleanse, which is designed to release toxins only in the colon, not the toxins stored in our fat cells.

WHY DOES NUTRITIONAL FASTING PRODUCE SUCH DRAMATIC RESULTS?

During my personal nutritional fasting experience, antioxidant botanicals, such as Aloe gel, licorice root, and ashwagandha root, supported liver detoxification and reduced my cravings. My body was consistently and sufficiently nourished with nutritious elements and ionic micro minerals and essential trace elements, instead of empty calories. Even when my body was immersed in a deep nutritional fasting day, I was continually satisfied. For the first time in my life, I was fortified with the appropriate amounts of vitamins, botanicals, and elements from the essential mineral suites–a need that extends far beyond just calories. This is a new paradigm in nutritional science.

After enlisting in this program, it forever changed my perceptions of the true meaning of health. I now know it is not the number of calories that matter in achieving a healthy lifestyle, but the makeup of nutrition that is contained within those calories. What our bodies really require are nutrient-dense super calories.

Though at the time I was completely amazed at these results, now I do not consider my story that unusual–the average weight loss for men and women is seven pounds in just 11 days, based on a clinical study of the nutritional approach that I used. This still remains a remarkable feat, as you know, if you have suffered through any diet and/or exercise program to lose only a pound a week, like I had previously.

The transformation I saw in my life motivated me to find out why this particular program worked and why every other diet I had tried had failed me every time I tried them. It is based on real nutritional science and revolutionary new nutritional approaches developed over more than 35 years ago.

When you apply a nutritional detox approach, it essentially expedites the three phases of detoxification in the body. First, the toxins stored in the body are metabolized along with breaking down harmful enzymes. This first process not only makes toxins water soluble; it also converts these toxins into molecules that are usually less toxic and safer for the body. As they are broken down, they can now easily be transported into the blood and into the kidneys, allowing the body to eliminate these toxins through urine. The second phase helps enzymes add water-soluble molecules onto the toxin, which breaks down the toxin again and makes it less toxic to the body and easy to eliminate through urine. The third phase helps to eliminate toxins from cells. This combination of the first two phases of detoxification collaborate to remove toxins from cells and prepare them for elimination the same ways as in phase one and two. We will cover this again later in the book.

WHEY PROTEIN'S CRITICAL ROLE IN WEIGHT MANAGEMENT

What is whey protein's critical role to our weight management, longevity, wellness, and our very existence in the toxic world we live in today? The whey protein in these "super shakes" is in a class by itself when compared to other sources of protein like meat, eggs, fish, soy, and many other sources. The right whey protein has very unique properties, some of which mimic mother's breast milk: humanity's first perfect food.

Whey shakes use extraordinary and uncommon raw, carefully selected, undenatured whey protein that can change the quality of your life and give you the ability to enhance your wellness potential and, specifically, your gene potential. Consuming these shakes provides you with incredible health benefits and energy that you cannot get from other foods or protein sources.

THE ROLE OF THERMOGENESIS IN WEIGHT LOSS

An important component to weight loss is thermogenesis. It occurs when a portion of dietary calories in excess of those required for immediate energy requirements are converted to heat, rather than stored as fat. When it comes to stimulating thermogenesis and satisfying appetite, it's well-known that dietary protein is king over carbohydrates and fats. The type of protein you choose is also critical.

There are two major types of milk protein: casein (usually referred to as milk protein) and whey. According to research published in 2011 in the *American Journal of Clinical Nutrition*, whey protein consumed at breakfast, lunch, and dinner proved more successful than either milk protein or soy protein for boosting fat burning and simultaneously reducing muscle loss.

The scientists conducted a double-blind, randomized, placebo-controlled study, measuring the thermic effect of meals high in whey, milk protein, or soy proteins, with a high carbohydrate meal as a control. They found that the total energy expenditure over 5.5 hours was greater after consuming the whey protein meal versus the other proteins, and all were significantly higher than the high-carbohydrate meal.

The thermic effect of food is a measurement of the amount of energy that is required for digestion and absorption and metabolism. Simply stated, the act of eating and digesting both brings in calories and burns them. Eating foods with a higher thermic effect can support weight management goals and, in the case of whey protein, even promote muscle growth.

More than just a metabolic measure, the thermic effect of foods reflects the rate that fats, proteins, and carbohydrates are broken down for energy in our bodies. The researchers explained the high thermic effect of whey protein might be due to the amino acid composition. Whey is high in leucine, a branched-chain amino acid, which has been shown to stimulate muscle protein synthesis and muscle maintenance.

In addition to boosting fat burning potential, a protein-rich diet also resulted in a much lower postprandial (occurring after a meal) glucose response than the carbohydrate control. We all know the feeling of an afternoon crash: eyes struggling to stay open, concentration drifting to thoughts of snuggling up in bed, and overall energy depletion. Glucose may be the body's main fuel source, but now a new study suggests that protein should be what we eat at lunch to help us stay awake and burn calories for the rest of the afternoon.

Orexin Burns Calories

University of Cambridge researchers compared the effects of different nutrients on neurons in mouse brains. Wakefulness and calorie burning are dependent on secretion of a neuropeptide, orexin. When neurons don't secrete enough orexin, sleepiness ensues—which can lead to fewer calories burned and more weight gained over time.

When the scientists measured the actions of protein (amino acids), carbohydrate (glucose) and fat (fatty acids) on the neurons, they found that the amino acids stimulated the cells to secrete orexin to a much greater extent than the other nutrients. In prior studies, the researchers found that orexin-secreting neurons are blocked by glucose. But when interactions between glucose and protein were looked at in this study, the researchers found that protein prevents glucose from blocking the orexin secretion. Lead researcher Denis Burdakov of the University of Cambridge Department of Pharmacology and Institute of Metabolic Science simply stated, "Electrical impulses emitted by orexin cells stimulate wakefulness and tell the body to burn calories."

This may help explain why people may feel particularly sleepy after eating meals rich in carbohydrates. Meals higher in protein and lower in total carbohydrates could help maintain alertness over the course of the day.

"What is exciting is to have a rational way to 'tune' select brain cells to be more or less active by deciding what food to eat. Not all brain cells are simply turned on by all nutrients, dietary composition is critical," said Burdakov.

For now, research suggests that if you have a choice between jam on toast or egg whites on toast, go for the latter!

Even though the two may contain the same number of calories, having a bit of protein will tell the body to burn more calories out of those consumed.

EXERCISE AND DIET LIMITATIONS

We are spending billions of dollars each year on diets that fail most of the time. The promise of weight loss is a great business, where you can have a 90 percent failure rate and the customers keep coming! What a mess. I was certainly part of this false hope that the ads portrayed.

In reality, I realized I was forcing myself to have hope, because even though I had extreme motivation to lose weight and be compliant, I had such limited success. I am not sure I could have continued on the diet and exercise program prescribed by my doctor, even though I was worried about my health.

Along with diet, exercise is peddled as the missing link to successful weight loss. Although exercise supports overall health and wellness, I was shocked to learn that many experts, as a result of research studies, believe it does not work, at least not as a lone strategy for losing weight.

2016 Study on Exercise and Its Limitations for Weight Loss

To give you some examples, a 2016 study published in the journal *Current Biology* measured the daily energy expenditure and activity levels of 332 adults over the course of a week. The scientists found that exercise alone isn't sufficient for weight loss, apparently because most human bodies reach a sort of plateau at which more vigorous activity fails to burn extra calories.

Earlier studies in *The British Journal of Sports Medicine* reached similar conclusions. One of the study researchers, Edward Melanson, PhD, an associate professor at the University of Colorado School of Medicine, explained a primary reason why exercise alone doesn't burn off weight and keep it off: "In a typical 30-minute exercise session, you are only burning 200 or 300 calories. You replace that with one bottle of Gatorade."

Mark Schauss, author of *Achieving Victory Over a Toxic World*, and an expert on laboratory testing and environmental health issues, explained the exercise quandary this way: "Exercise does not help lose weight in most people but only helps to not gain any pounds. This is somewhat profound and makes you realize that if someone truly wants to lose weight, it is by improving the resting metabolic rate that you can hope to succeed. If toxins can (and they do) impair this process, we need to discover ways to improve that mechanism through detoxification and toxin avoidance."

While maintaining an active lifestyle with an exercise routine has proven to help people live longer and healthier, it is only one small part of the key to weight loss. After two months of killing myself in the gym with routines that most people would never attempt, I had lost only eight pounds. There was no way I would have kept up that extreme exercise routine with so little to show for it. And yet, in popular dieting programs that is hailed as a great goal.

Not for me anymore. No way, no how, and I am never going back to diet and exercise as the solution for weight loss and extreme health now that I am aware of a revolutionary new approach.

The Real Benefits of Exercise

Please note that the authors of this book exercise on a regular basis and in no way, are stating that exercise does not have huge benefits. The point is that those who believe that exercise is one of the sole solutions to weight loss as is stated above is false. However, exercise is an integral part of maintaining a healthy life style. There are tremendous benefits from a cardiovascular stand point. It has been shown that just walking 15 to 30 minutes a day is a very helpful contributor for our overall health. It has also been shown in several journals that resistance training can help to change fat/lean muscle composition. Almost any kind of exercise can help you to relieve stress, in addition to strengthening your body. Consider exercise an adjunct strategy, not a main course strategy, for losing pounds and keeping them off.

The US Department of Health and Human Services recommends at least 150 minutes of moderate aerobic exercise or 75 minutes of vigorous aerobic exercise per week.[7] The agency also recommends strength training at least twice per week.

Moderate aerobic exercises include brisk walking, swimming, and even mowing the front lawn. Vigorous aerobic exercise includes running and aerobic dancing. Then there is strength or resistance training, which generally involves weights or machines. As always, it is recommended that you consult with your health professional before embarking on any exercise or nutritional program.

YOGA'S EFFECTS ON WEIGHT LOSS

As a form of exercise, yoga has been underestimated when it comes to having an impact on the body's ability to lose weight. Medical researcher and practicing yogi, Alan Kristal, DPH, MPH, completed a medical study in 2005 on the weight-loss effects of yoga. Kristal led a trial involving 15,500 healthy, middle-aged men and women. All participants completed a survey recalling their physical activity (including yoga) and their weight between the ages of 45 and 55. Practicing yoga was defined as at least one 30-minute session per week for four or more years.

The results, according to Kristal, indicated, "Those practicing yoga who were overweight to start with, lost about 5 pounds during the same time period; those not practicing yoga gained 14 pounds."[8] The reasons why yoga worked in this way are not as clear. Many conjecture that an increase in mindfulness might have the biggest impact. The way in which we bring awareness to our eating practices can lead to a letting go of destructive eating habits and bring healthy eating practices in a way that is easeful and sustainable.

Yoga contains as many styles of yoga as shoes in a shoe store, and each are as different as high-heeled pumps are from snow boots. Some claim that styles of yoga such as Power Yoga are aerobic, due to the coupling of actively flowing through poses with breath, and the increased oxygen of the added focus on breath.

Others, such as Judith Hanson Lasater, a leading expert in Restorative Yoga, who assisted in the design of the yoga program used in a study of yoga and metabolic syndrome at the University of California at San Francisco, suggests that through deep rest we can reduce stress. As we've covered before, an increase in stress hormones can encourage the body to store fat around the belly. So through a decrease in stress, one could see a reduction in the pattern of abdominal weight gain.

If you are using yoga for weight loss, here are a few things to consider:

- Find a class or video that you can practice with where you find you are challenged yet are encouraged to honor your body and rest or come out of poses as needed.

- Set specific goals and track and measure results. For instance, commit to practice yoga three to five days a week for one hour. Add specific classes to your schedule, or set aside time each week to practice with a yoga DVD or yoga video online. At the end of each week, measure your progress and reevaluate your practice for the next week and recommit. Start out with a goal for the next 40 days, which is the time required to shift a habit.

- Find a yoga practice that challenges both your body and mind. Allow your practice to be pleasurable and seek out ways it can be more pleasurable for you. Women's bodies respond chemically to pleasure in a way that is motivating, so they are more likely to do things that give them pleasure.

- Combine your yoga practice with nutritional fasting.

Yoga and Metabolic Types

In the community of yoga practitioners, one population swears by yoga for weight loss, as they have experienced dramatic results. Another group of practitioners has experienced weight gain. In some cases, weight gain can be attributed to following dietary guidelines that are in conflict with an individual's bio-individuality, specifically their metabolic type. Metabolic types include: Protein type, Carbohydrate type, Mixed type, or Variable type, with Protein and Carbohydrate types, being the most common.

For example, protein and fats to carbohydrate ratios for Protein types are 70 percent protein and fats and 30 percent carbohydrates, and for Carbohydrate types, they are 50 percent protein and fats and 50 percent carbohydrates. Protein types do well on dense protein such as buffalo, beef, lamb, tuna, and wild salmon. Carbohydrate types do well on lighter proteins such as quinoa and light, white fish such as tilapia and sole. Both do well on whey protein, especially for increasing lean muscle mass.

Some yoga traditions enact a pressure, or sometimes a requirement, to adopt a vegetarian or vegan lifestyle. While this works for some individuals and they may lose weight, for others this conflicts with the physiological way that their bodies naturally process food (fast oxidizers versus slow oxidizers).

When people eat in conflict with their metabolic type, they often gain weight and have low energy. When they eat in sync with their metabolic type, they tend to release fat and gain muscle toward their ideal body composition and have abundant energy. Someone who is a Protein type who is eating vegan or vegetarian may struggle to have 70 percent of their diet come from protein. Also, they will generally be sourcing protein from less dense protein sources. If someone is a Protein type who is also vegan or vegetarian, it becomes increasingly important to have a reliable source of high-quality protein to add to their existing nutrition as well as options that are easy to carry and consume when on the go.

YOGA FOR TO HELP THOSE WHO ARE OVERWEIGHT—A MINDFUL PRACTICE

The following exercise can be used as a visualization technique while you are in the midst of your yoga routine. It can be very helpful.

Imagine yourself standing in front of your most common obstacle regarding overeating. Some examples of this might include pulling into the drive thru at your favorite fast food chain, standing in front of the vending machine at work, picking up the phone to call pizza delivery, or standing in the candy or snack aisle at the grocery store. See all the images your eyes might see. Smell the smells. Hear the sounds. Feel the temperatures, textures, and sensations on your skin.

First witness your current pattern. For instance, see yourself place the order at the drive thru, pick it up at the window, and park and eat in your car.

Now feel how your body feels. What do you see, smell, hear, and feel? Do a body scan. Start with your feet. Observe your legs, pelvic area, abdominal area, torso, arms, hands, shoulders, neck, head, and face. Do you feel cold or hot, empty or full or over full, tight or relaxed, soft or hard, bloated or gassy? Do you feel any sensations of pain or numbness? Note all these sensations or it may be powerful to speak them or write them down.

Now close your eyes again. Visualize yourself in the same situation, standing in front of your most common obstacle regarding overeating. Ask yourself what you see, smell, hear, and feel.

Now take three breaths, elongating each one. In addition, let each exhale be twice as long as the inhale. For example, on the first breath, inhale to a count of 3; exhale to a count of 6. For the second breath, inhale to a count of 4; exhale to a count of 8. For the third breath, inhale to a count of 5; exhale to a count of 10.

Engaging in this practice can help you to overcome some of your most challenging food temptations, as you begin to realize that certain foods do not actually make your body feel good and you learn a more effective way to avoid them.

*   *   *

In chapter one we explained why nutritional fasting and yoga can both help to eliminate your body's toxicity and now you know that they can also play an important role as an intervention in the overweight category of the TDOS Syndrome. Consuming a nutrient-dense diet not only keeps you feeling satisfied and prevents hunger but also provides your body with the necessary vitamins and essential minerals to maintain energy and operate efficiently, burning fat and destroying the toxins that can lead to overweight. While exercise can help alleviate stress, a major component in TDOS, it cannot be relied on as the sole solution for tackling overweight, however yoga appears to have more success because it increases mindfulness of destructive eating habits. In the next chapter, we'll examine its specific effect on stress as well as other successful stress-management techniques.

Chapter Four

Stress Interventions

The following is a summary of the problem of stress (as identified in our book *The TDOS Syndrome*):

1. Chronic stress wears many faces. It can be disguised as anxiety, depression, fatigue, loss of motivation, or insecurity, and it evolves over time to become a major factor in the onset of many disease processes, including the acceleration of aging.

2. We need a certain minimum amount of stress, and the hormone cortisol that it produces, to remain functional and activated in setting and achieving goals. There is a tipping point, however, and most people don't know the warning signs to indicate when the tip-over into chronic stress has been initiated.

3. The human body requires specific nutrients to offset stress, and, because we face a massive nutritional deficiency in our diets, those nutrients are not available to us and, as a result, chronic stress worsens.

4. Chronic stress is expensive to individuals and society. The Centers for Disease Control estimates that 80 percent of all health-care dollars are spent on stress-related issues, and the American Medical Association estimates that stress causes 80 to 85 percent of all health problems.

5. Some of the most common stress-related health problems are stomach problems like ulcers, but stress also causes high

blood pressure, heart disease, asthma, allergies, cancer, and even headaches.

6. Chronic stress, releasing chronic levels of cortisol, sends the body a message *not* to burn fat. This chronic stress and chronically elevated cortisol are crucial factors in our inability to lose fat and weight, contributing to the epidemic of obesity. Even the *thought* of losing weight can be stressful. The more you try to diet, the more stress you feel, and the more cortisol that goes into your system, essentially turning off the body's ability to burn fat.

7. Research has shown that overweight people secrete large levels of stress hormones after eating a meal, making them more susceptible to cardiovascular disease and type 2 diabetes. The act of eating, in and of itself, raises stress levels in the bodies of overweight people by 50 percent and more, above stress hormones released by normal weight people.

8. Some chemical toxins interact with stress to produce synergistic effects on health, either triggering illness and disease, or weakening the immune system to make illness and disease more possible.

STRESS MANAGEMENT WITHOUT DRUGS

We don't want to entirely get rid of our fight-or-flight stress response. In fact, acute fear can be a good thing. It allows us to quickly respond to danger. Even anxiety, which is a notch down, can be helpful at the right dose. Too little stress, and we might not accomplish as much, but too much can be harmful. Having the correct balance of stress motivates us to make changes and do useful things.

Everyone has a stress signature, which is a certain way someone's body feels when he or she is stressed, and how that person stores his or her tension. Developing an awareness of the stress signature is a key to relieving tension because awareness allows for the release of it.

As long as tension and anxiety remain under the surface, it is difficult to induce relaxation.

In the same way that you have a stress signature, you also have a relaxation signature. That is, certain elements will relax you faster than others. You also have stressors that may cause you to tense up more than others.

One of my goals in writing this book is to provide you with the methods, strategies, and techniques to help you find your relaxation signature. Once you have found it, you will find it easier to extract elements that will instantly provide you with relaxation.

USE EXERCISE WITH OTHER STRESS REDUCTION TECHNIQUES

An effective way to discharge or resolve the fight-or-flight response is with exercise. Studies reveal that regular workouts increase stress resistance, decrease anxiety, diminish depression, and generally leave people more cheerful. Physically active children report happier moods and less depression, and they cope better with stress than children who are not as active. Even middle-aged people who have been sedentary for years do almost as well as people who have been active all their lives.

As a supplement to physical activity, there are many science-proven—and natural—methods for stress relief, and we'll examine them in this chapter.

YOGA'S EFFECT ON STRESS

Scientific evidence supports yoga as an antidote to stress. Among many benefits, yoga relaxes the nervous system, which has an effect on the body's stress response.

According to studies by the Trauma Research Institute in Boston, Massachusetts, yoga reduces heart rate variability (HRV), a co-factor in stress. Other studies have shown mindfulness practices, such as yoga, to be linked to de-activation of the default mode network (DMN).

The DMN is the brain system that is active during mind-wandering and worrisome thoughts, which can increase stress.

Methods such as yoga train the brain to respond to stress differently and can improve our memory, focus, and executive functions like problem solving, planning, organization, and decision making. One can imagine both the primary and peripheral benefits of improvement in those areas.

Practicing mindfulness techniques, such as yoga, may lead to less impulsive reactions and behaviors, more awareness of the thoughts and emotions that drive our behavior, and a decrease in disempowered choices.

COGNITIVE BEHAVIORAL THERAPY (CBT)

This technique can be an effective way to reduce stress by allowing you to examine your own irrational thought patterns that produce anxiety. These patterns may include the following:

- *Catastrophizing*–This involves exaggerating the harmful effect of events that happen to you. Example: When your boss offers mild criticism, you're sure you'll be fired.

- *Over-generalizing*–Here you are interpreting one unpleasant situation as part of an endless pattern. Example: When you are turned down for a date, you feel rejected by the whole world.

- *Mental filtering*–Here you focus on the negative while screening out the positive. Example: You obsess about your B in history class when all your other grades were A's.

A typical CBT approach to overcoming irrational thought patterns involves this sequence of steps:

- *Identify Sources of Stress*—One approach is keeping a diary to record daily events and activities, recording which activities trigger anger or anxiety.

- *Question the Sources of Stress*—Individuals ask themselves the following questions: Do these stressful activities meet my goals or someone else's? Have I taken on tasks that I can reasonably accomplish? Which tasks are under my control and which ones aren't?

- *Restructuring Priorities and Adding Stress-Reducing Activities*—This is where the client shifts his or her focus from stress-producing to stress-reducing activities. Examples might include: Take time for recreation prior to shopping for groceries.

THE QUIETING REFLEX

Another simple stress-management technique is The Quieting Reflex, developed by Dr. Charles Stroebel[9]—a technique you can use to relax in just six seconds. Here's how it works:

1. Think about something you fear.

2. Smile. According to Dr. Stroebel, this breaks up tension in the face.

3. Affirm, "I can keep a calm body and an alert mind."

4. Take an easy deep breath.

5. Open your mouth slightly to relax the jaw.

6. Visualize heaviness and warmth moving throughout your body.

MEDITATION CAN LOWER BLOOD PRESSURE

Mindfulness is a form of meditation that trains people to remain in the present moment, rather than thinking about the future or the past. Mindfulness meditation techniques are designed to help you stay alert and in the present moment, which can be a place of tranquility, as opposed to the past or future, where there are often strong emotions and conflicting thoughts. This redirection of brain activity from your thoughts and worries to your senses disrupts the stress response, prompting relaxation. It also helps promote an emotional and sensual appreciation of simple pleasures. One book I often recommend for new meditators is 8 *Minute Meditation: Quiet Your Mind. Change Your Life* by Victor Davich.

Some mindfulness techniques involve heightening awareness of the immediate surrounding environment. Here, you choose a routine activity like washing dishes and concentrate on the feel of the water and dishes. If the mind begins to think about the past or future, or fills with unformed thoughts or worries, redirect it gently back to the physical activity of washing the dishes.

Meditation can be used are for physical relaxation, mental relaxation, pain control, bringing order to brain frequencies, creating a more even emotional state, enhanced creativity, and even reducing heart disease. Upon entering a meditative state, you become more relaxed. In this relaxation, the body begins to heal itself.

Each type of meditation technique has many things in common, such as repetition. You can alter your brain frequency by silently repeating a word, phrase, or sound. This is known as a mantra. The mantra is the basis of Transcendental Meditation. It entails repeating one word over and over, until you enter an altered state.

The more spiritual and true the sound, the better for spiritual enlightenment, but in reality, any sound will work. For example, "Om Namah Shivaya" in Sanskrit means, "I bow to the divine self within." In Siddha Yoga, this is repeated while sitting quietly. After a few minutes, you get into the harmony and musical sound of the mantra.

To end the meditation, you can say to yourself: "At the count of five I will be wide awake, feeling fine, and in perfect health." Then count slowly from 1 to 3. On the count of 3 say to yourself, "at the count of 5, I will be wide awake feeling fine and in perfect health." Then count 4 and 5, and say, "Eyes open, feeling fine, and in perfect health, feeling better than before."

A SIMPLE MEDITATION USING NUMBERS

Find a comfortable sitting position. Uncross your hands and feet. Close your eyes and relax. Tell yourself that you are going to mentally repeat and visualize the numbers 10 to 1: Take a deep breath and while exhaling, mentally repeat and visualize the number 10 several times. Take another deep breath and while exhaling mentally repeat and visualize the number 9 several times. Do these for each descending number until you reach the number 1. After you reach the number 1, say to yourself, "I am now relaxed physically and mentally. Each time I practice this I will get even more relaxed than I am right now." While you are relaxed, you can visualize passive scenes or review projects that you may be working on. You may notice that it is easier to find solutions to these projects while meditating."

HEART MATH INSTITUTE STRESS STRATEGIES

You may have never heard of this science research group, but it's beginning to have a profound effect on how we understand the relationship between our heart and our mind. The Heart Math Institute describes its origins and stress-related technologies and strategies this way on their website:

"Heart Math was founded in 1991 to help individuals, organizations and the global community incorporate the heart's intelligence into their day-to-day experience of life. We do this by connecting heart and science in ways that empower people to greatly reduce stress, build resilience, and unlock their natural intuitive guidance for making better choices. Since our inception we have been developing and delivering research-based, practical, and reliable tools and technologies that enable people to align and connect their heart, mind and emotions to produce transformative outcomes—with more flow and less stress."

Based on its 18 years of scientific research on stress and behaviors, the Heart Math Institute developed both technologies and practical exercises for stress relief. For example, in a 2013 issue of the science journal *Applied Psychophysiology and Biofeedback*, scientists with the Institute reported how diaphragmatic breathing, at six breaths per minute, could quickly diminish stress.

By regulating your breath, you learn to also regulate the release of the stress hormone, cortisol, particularly during and after emotionally challenging situations.

Here is a simple one-minute exercise:

1. Place a hand over your heart area and focus your attention there.

2. Pretend you are breathing through your heart area.

3. Breathe slowly and gently until your breathing is smooth and balanced, with a natural rhythm.

4. Summon appreciation or gratitude for someone or something in your life.

5. Sustain this feeling with heart focus, heart breathing, and heart feeling, doing so for one minute.

For more information, visit www.heartmath.org.

A TDOS *SOLUTION PROVIDER*:
DIRECT NEUROFEEDBACK AND STRESS RELIEF
FROM THE DUBIN CLINIC

Direct neurofeedback is an emerging technology that sends a brief (within seconds), tiny signal back to the brain. This signal causes a slight fluctuation in brainwaves and enables the brain to get out of frozen or stuck patterns. It allows the brain to reorganize itself, like rebooting a frozen computer. Patients of The Dubin Clinic claim they usually notice significant change within the first few sessions.

To share insights on this powerful therapy, I've asked my good friend and colleague, David Dubin, MD, to provide his observations, after years of work in this field. Dr. Dubin graduated from The University of Medicine and Dentistry of New Jersey and then completed a residency in Emergency Medicine. He subsequently worked as an Associate Clinical Professor of Outpatient Medicine at Boston University. After a career of more than ten years in Emergency Medicine, Dr. Dubin founded Cambridge Medical Consultants, providing Occupational and Environmental Medicine consulting to hospitals and corporations.

Disenchanted with treating patients primarily with medication, Dr. Dubin researched neurofeedback and found significant improvement in his own brain physiology. He began treating patients and saw rapid, meaningful, and often dramatic results. Equally remarkable, he found these changes to be enduring.

His experience echoed recent research in neuroplasticity, demonstrating new possibilities for growth and change within the brain. He soon decided to dedicate his career exclusively to the practice of direct neurofeedback, a very particular form of neurofeedback. He founded The Dubin Clinic, where he provides direct neurofeedback to adults, adolescents, and children.

Dr. Dubin's Direct Neurofeedback Technology*

Traditional Neurofeedback, also known as EEG bio-feedback, has been around for more than thirty years. It is a form of training the brain so its brainwaves have "healthier patterns." Sensors are placed on the scalp, and these sensors measure electrical activity of the brain. It is exactly the same as an EKG, or electrocardiogram, which has sensors over the heart, measuring its electrical activity. This information from the brain goes along wires to a small amplifier and then on to a computer. That information can be seen in the form of brainwaves, and it is called an EEG, or electroencephalogram. With neuro-feedback, the patient watches his brainwaves and tries to influence them by receiving real-time feedback about what his brain is doing. The feedback is often in the form of a game. There might be a spaceship, for example, and when the brainwaves are going in the desired pattern the spaceship moves. If the brainwaves go in an undesirable pattern, the spaceship slows down or stops. The patient is receiving live feedback, and through this he learns to train his brain. While a great deal more research needs to be done, studies show that neurofeedback can be helpful in, among other things: anxiety, depression, ADHD, autism, concussions, and, particularly for this chapter, stress. Traditional neurofeedback typically takes 40 to 60 sessions and results do not usually begin right away.

Direct Neurofeedback is a cutting-edge brain technology that is actually quite different than traditional neurofeedback. As before, sensors on the scalp track the brain's electrical activity and then travel via wires to an amplifier and on to a computer. Now, however, a tiny electromagnetic signal is sent back to the brain.

A patient cannot feel or even notice this signal—it is imperceptible. Its strength is far less than that of a cell phone. This signal causes a slight fluctuation in brainwaves and allows the brain to get out of rigid, stuck neural patterns and reorganize itself. It's like rebooting a frozen computer.

The patient is completely passive and does not have to do anything. The whole procedure typically only takes about ten minutes. The patient does not interact with the computer monitor. Direct neurofeedback does not train the brain like biofeedback or traditional neurofeedback. Rather, it interrupts dysfunctional patterns. It "dis-entrains" the brain.

The signal is not directed at specific dysfunctional areas of the brain; the effects are global. A useful metaphor is that the signal is like gently shaking a palm tree that has one stuck branch. The healthy, flexible branches wave in the wind and then return to their original position. The one stuck branch, however, is freed up.

The brain responds very rapidly to this form of therapy. In fact, most patients begin to experience some initial improvement in the first session. Initial changes are temporary, typically lasting from a few hours to a few days. With additional sessions, the effects last longer. Also, the baseline improves, so that even when the effect of a treatment wears off, the starting point is better than prior to starting. For most disorders it takes about 15–20 sessions for the benefits to endure.

The central nervous system (CNS) consists of our brain and spinal cord. The nerves from the spinal cord on out to the rest of the body are called the peripheral nervous system (PNS). One part of the PNS acts as an accelerator (the sympathetic nervous system, or "fight or flight" response). A second part acts as a brake to the nervous system. This is the parasympathetic nervous system, or the "rest and digest" response). With anxiety, PTSD (post-traumatic stress disorder), chronic anxiety, and more, the accelerator is pressed down to the floor but no one is stepping on the brakes. As a result, the nervous system is in constant overdrive, and this leads to **chronic stress and anxiety**.

There are plenty of statistics showing the negative influence chronic stress and anxiety have on our health. Forty-three percent of all adults suffer adverse health effects from stress. Seventy-five to 90 percent of all doctor's office visits are for stress-related complaints. These may include heart disease, asthma, diabetes, fibromyalgia, headaches, depression, anxiety, gastrointestinal problems.

It is undeniable that chronic stress and anxiety have profound and pervasive effects on our health. When someone receives direct neurofeedback, change is usually obvious. There is frequently a deep sigh and the rate of breathing slows down. Her face and entire musculature relax, she talks less and fidgets less, and even the muscles of the voice box relax, causing her voice to become a little deeper. The stress and anxiety simply melt away, because the foot is off the accelerator and the brake is in use. It's a huge relief for the patient and extremely gratifying to me.

*None of these statements have been evaluated by the FDA. The comments and observations printed here are those of Dr. David Dubin. For additional information on Direct Neurofeedback, visit www.thedubinclinic.com, and www.DirectNeurofeedback. com. For more information on neurofeedback research, visit http://www.isnr.org/ resources/comprehensive-bibliography.cfm

NATURE CAN HELP US REDUCE STRESS

In addition to meditation and other stress management techniques, we also have access to what nature provides us in the form of natural botanicals, proven to assist in the lowering and management of stress. These botanicals are a huge part of The New Health Conversation and the TDOS Solution.

We need an offensive plan against stress based on preventive interventions. The strategy includes utilization of multiple solutions and nutrients working together to diminish the effects of stress and its by-products.

Shilajit—A Miraculous Ingredient from Nepal

Shilajit is an extruded material that is pressed out from layers of rock in the mountains of Nepal and other high-range mountains. It is composed of humus and organic plant material that has been trapped and compressed by layers of rock, under billions of pounds of pressure. Humus is formed when soil microorganisms decompose from plant material into bio-rich nutrients and elements usable by plants. Plants are the source of all our food, and humus is the source of plant food.

Due to microbial action and the tremendous pressure from the weight of the mountains, Shilajit was transformed into a dense, viscous, mineral-rich mass, possibly the richest organic mass ever created on the planet. Shilajit is revered by the Nepalese as a very strong destroyer of weakness and builder of health.

The trapped layers of Shilajit became exposed due to the freezing winters, hot summer sun, and the expansion and contraction of the mountain range. Shilajit will "flow" out from between the cliff cracks in the layers of rock during the summer, when the mountain temperatures rise. Shilajit quickly dries to a soft, breakable stone-like black mass and can be consumed as a dissolvable powder or liquid.

For thousands of years, the Nepalese scaled the mountain cliffs, repelling down to collect Shilajit, their medicine of choice they came to depend on. Shilajit is used today in Ayurvedic health practices. The Nepalese find that its strength is better if mixed with goat's milk and honey. It seems to give them more energy, relieve digestive problems, increase sex drive, and improve memory and cognition. The beneficial stress-protective effect of adaptogens is related to the regulation of homeostasis via mechanisms of action associated with the hypothalamic-pituitary-adrenal axis and the regulation of key mediators of the stress response, such as molecular chaperones, stress-activated c-Jun N-terminal protein kinase, fork head box O transcription factor, cortisol, and nitric oxide (NO).

Scientists now know why the effects are more profound when mixed in the ancient tonic. Honey and goat's milk contain enzymes that neutralize certain unwanted molecules that are caught up in the mass. Today's Shilajit undergoes a purification process that replicates the one used by ancient medicine men.

The therapeutic actions of raw Shilajit vary, according to the region of origin and mountain range. Similar substances contain humic and fulvic acids, but true Shilajit has a unique therapeutic, bioactive ingredient that is not present in other "Shilajit-like" substances.

The authenticity and therapeutic quality of Shilajit can be identified through laboratory analysis. The primary active ingredients in Shilajit are fulvic acids, dibenzo alpha pyrones, and humins. Humic acids and fulvic acids are small molecules that act as carriers for the dibenzo alpha pyrones. They carry other nutrients with them as well.

While there are several areas that the raw material is collected from, the highest levels of therapeutic ingredients come from specific areas in the Himalayan Mountains in Nepal at 14,000 to 15,900 feet above sea level. Historic records report that these "sacred" mountains produce the best Shilajit.

High quality shilajit can be purchased from specialty supplement companies online.

Stress-Fighting Adaptogens

Russian scientist Dr. Israel Brekhman spent 15 years of research on adaptogens, which Brekhman and his colleagues defined as natural plant substances that:

1. Increase the body's ability to cope with internal and external stresses.

2. Exhibit stimulating effects leading to increased working capacity and mental performance under stressful and fatigue-inducing conditions.

3. Normalize the functions of the body.

4. Are entirely safe and have no negative side effects.

His research on adaptogens introduced formulas that promote health by helping people cope with everyday stress, maintain high levels of energy, and free the body from fatigue. While all adaptogens are restorative to the body's stress response and capacity to perform, certain combinations studied by Brekhman are better suited for the exclusive purpose of boosting performance and fighting fatigue.

When selecting the best nutrient rich drink to reduce stress, you will want to make sure it contains adaptogens.[10] This unique cocktail of powerful adaptogens, essential mineral groups, and trace elements, in drink form, can work synergistically with your body to protect you against the harmful effects of stress, while also promoting healthy aging.

* * *

We often fail to recognize what a powerful effect stress has on our bodies. It is a critical component in the TDOS Syndrome. Thankfully, there are numerous ways to counteract stress, including physical exercise, yoga, cognitive behavioral therapy, meditation, direct neurofeedback, and more. Even certain plant substances have the ability to reduce our stress. In part II we'll take a more in-depth look at nutritional fasting and exactly how to implement this incredible tool into your life.

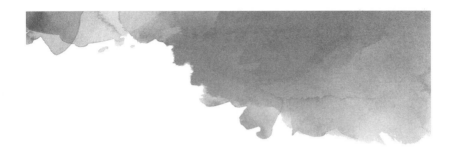

PART TWO

Following the Program

Chapter Five

The Healing Practice of Nutritional Fasting

Fasting has been a traditional healing practice for thousands of years, intended to help enhance many of the body's internal detoxification and cleansing systems.

Reduced food intake allows the body to purify itself through rest and renewal, while the use of botanicals, such as Aloe gel, licorice root, and ashwagandha root, contain bio-active components to support the liver—the body's natural detoxifier.

Age-old traditions of fasting have now been combined with modern technologies into new nutritional approaches that provide nourishment to the body, in order to efficiently deal with daily toxic loads and stresses. In my own quest to detoxify my body, I used the TDOS Solution's suggestion of an Aloe vera juice drink, utilizing the inner heart filet of the *Aloe* plant, and enhanced with the "Mineral Suites." This drink supports the liver, immune system, and overall cellular health, by utilizing a combination of vitamins, herbal teas, and other botanical ingredients.

BEGINNING A NUTRITIONAL FASTING LIFESTYLE

I'm going to outline the basics for how to start the program. You will continue this until you have reached your goals, and then you can go on a simple maintenance program.

Please note: When we refer to "Super Shake Days," we are referring to the raw, carefully selected, undenatured whey protein that is available in England, Italy, Switzerland, Germany, New Zealand, Canada, Australia, and many other countries in the world, and even in the US if you look hard enough for it. More information regarding protein and Super Shakes will be provided in chapter eight.

We also are referring to the Super Vegan Shakes. We provide you with both Shake recipes and or show you what to look for if you are purchasing them commercially from a fulfillment company.

The optimal nutritional fasting protocol is as follows:

1. Two to 4 days of Super Shake Days = Intermittent Caloric reduction

2. Then two days of Deep Nutritional Fasting Days = 48-hour nutritional fasting

3. Five to seven days of Super Shake Days = intermittent caloric restriction

4. Two days of Deep Nutritional Fasting Days = 48-hour nutritional fasting

5. Five to seven days of Feast Days = reduced caloric restriction

6. Two days of Deep Nutritional Fasting Days = 48-hour nutritional fasting

7. Keep repeating five to seven days of Super Shakes and two days of Deep Nutritional Fasting until you reach your desired goals.

The terms "Super Shake Days," "Nutritional Fasting," and Super Shake "Feast" Days will be explained in the following pages, and I will share some of my experiences with nutritional fasting.

What Is a Super Shake Day?

You start with two Super Shake days (intermittent caloric reduction without nutrient reduction) at the beginning of the program to prepare the body to take advantage of the Nutritional Fasting days. Your body will burn fat during these first two Super Shake days, as you also cut out unnecessary toxins, such as caffeine, sugars, diet sodas, and alcohol. We also suggest avoiding all processed foods and simple carbohydrates. Grains and non-pasteurized dairy is allowed on these days.

Simply drink a Super Shake for breakfast and dinner, and eat a healthy, 400–600 calorie meal of your choice of healthy food for lunch. You will be eating "real" healthy food for lunch. We usually suggest eating a lean piece of protein like chicken or fish. The rule of thumb is the piece of protein should be about the size of your fist. We also suggest vegetables and the greener they are the better. Additional recipes are included in chapter eight. You should also consider chewable whey-based mini meals and a combination of vitamins, botanicals, and essential elements from the mineral suites that can be purchased in health food stores or found online.

During this time, it is important to consume a minimum of eight 8-ounce glasses of water each day. To get the most out of the nutritional fasting experience, it is recommended that you drink half your body weight in number of ounces of water a day. For example, if you weigh 140 pounds, you should be consuming a minimum of 70 ounces of water daily. Water is an integral part of any nutritional fasting program, and drinking the necessary amount of water is an important habit to maintain smooth functioning within the body.

Be advised that water cannot be replaced with the small amounts contained in tea, soda as well as diet drinks. Pure water is the life-blood of the body and a main vehicle for carrying nutrients. It also disposes of the body's waste and facilitates detoxification processes. Every day through urination, perspiration, and respiration, we lose the equivalent of at least 64 ounces of water. To replenish this supply, we must drink substantial amounts of clean, purified water.

Nutritional Fasting Days

After increasing your water intake and allowing your body to assimilate nutritional fasting nutrients during the first two Super Shake days, you are ready to begin your first two days of Nutritional Fasting.

During the TDOS Solutions' nutritional fast, all Nutritional Fasting days are the same. Solid food is replaced with a super Aloe vera-based mineral drink (we call it liquid nutrition) that you can select where your fulfillment company should only use low-temperature spray-dried organic Aloe vera (see recipe below). This drink should either contain the necessary essential minerals or they should be added as a supplement along with the drink. In addition, you will consume a whey protein wafer or vegan wafer and a super vitamins and botanicals that contains ingredients (we listed above as to what to include) proven to help the body naturally cleanse.

During your Nutritional Fasting Days, you consume four ounces of the Super Aloe Vera Mineral Drink four times a day, six to eight of the nutritional whey mini-meals, and two super vitamin capsules. Because the Aloe vera, mini-meals, and super vitamin will flood your body with massive amounts of nutrients, botanicals, fats, and proteins, you shouldn't experience hunger, even without solid foods.

Some may experience what we call positive cleansing symptoms. These symptoms range from enjoyable and productive to the not so pleasant but experiencing these symptoms is proof positive that your body is in fact detoxing itself. Detox symptoms range from sound sleeping and mental clarity and weight loss to not so desirable symptoms ranging from headaches and fatigue as well as constipation and diarrhea. Whether they are helping to give you the best night of sleep in years, or have you running to the bathroom, the body has begun to naturally detox itself and in the long run, you will feel better all around.

Feast Days: Add Another Healthy Meal for Dinner

A Feast day is a Super Shake (whey or vegan protein shake) day during which you get to eat and enjoy dinner. Basically, the solution slightly changes as you consume a shake for breakfast, a healthy lunch of 400 to 600 calories, a healthy dinner containing 400 to 600 calories, and a shake about an hour after dinner for dessert. This makes the solution so much easier, as you can eat dinner with your family, friends, or significant other. That is why we call them Feast Days.

WHAT DOES A NUTRITIONAL FAST FEEL LIKE?

In the first 24 hours of Nutritional Fasting–while solid food is not consumed–the body uses up the sugar and glycogen stored in the liver and begins producing growth hormones to trigger fat burning and support lean muscle mass. Though the body begins its fat-burning processes on the first Nutritional Fasting day, by the end of the second day, excess sugar and carbohydrates stored in the liver have been used up, and maximum fat burning has been achieved. This is where the glutathione stored from the shakes and the polysaccharides from the Aloe vera begin naturally breaking down the toxins and making them water soluble.

The *body* is the source of all this detoxification because it is being supplied with these specific nutrients (toxin hunters). The body begins to burn off this excess fat (containing obesogens), causing it to shed pounds and inches quickly and safely. Throughout the Nutritional Fasting Solution, the body continues to increase levels of growth hormone to build muscle as the fat is released.

HOW DETOXIFICATION AND WEIGHT LOSS OCCUR

While I was on the Nutritional Fasting Solution, I consumed the super raw, carefully selected, undenatured whey protein shakes and chewable mini-meals that are packed with the same whey protein that is in the carefully selected shakes. These low-calorie mini-meals helped curb my hunger by providing small amounts of proteins, fats, and carbohydrates throughout the day. This kept my body in balance and prevented an afternoon crash of energy.

These mini-meals (wafers) maintained an overall nutritional balance in my body. The proteins supported lean muscle development, while the carbohydrates broke down into glucose, keeping my brain sharp, and the ionic essential trace minerals kept me fully nourished.

These nutritionally dense mini-meals should contain organic coconut oil, which is needed to slow down the release of glucose, maintain the body's fat-burning processes, and stimulate metabolism firings (speeds up metabolism and fat burning).

QUICK REFERENCE FOR MINI-MEAL INGREDIENTS

2–4 grams of undenatured whey protein, lecithin, silica, flax seed, chromium amino acid chelate. These snacks also need a few grams of sugar as well as up to 4 grams of carbohydrates and a minimal amount of fat. This is due to the fact that you want a mini-meal that is balanced according to the body's needs.

The last component in the nutritional fasting approach formula is what I like to refer to as The Super Nutrients Mix, a combination of nutrients, and cleansing herbs (listed in Quick Reference Box below) to assist the body in burning fat without stimulants. The Super Vitamin capsule naturally invigorates the body to maintain energy throughout the day while on the nutritional fast. In addition, you should take the essential macro minerals and micro minerals, and a variety of natural ingredients, including apple cider vinegar, green tea leaf extract, niacin, cinnamon-dried bark, and cayenne pepper.

QUICK REFERENCE FOR SUPER NUTRIENTS MIX COMBINATION OF INGREDIENTS

The Super Nutrients Mix should include ingredients that help stimulate metabolism, such as green tea extract, cinnamon, niacin, apple cider vinegar, cayenne pepper, and black pepper.

These natural nutrients ensure that the body is constantly satisfied with pure nourishment, even on a low-calorie diet. (Keep in mind that this capsule is for appetite support and not for appetite suppression.)

During my first Nutritional Fasting day, I was only ingesting liquid nutrition in the Super Aloe Vera Mineral Drink, Mini-Meals, and Super Vitamins, nutrients, cleansing herbs and drinking half my body weight in ounces of water. It surprised me that my body was fed and satisfied with massive amounts of this liquid nutrition. This happened because my body had all the necessary nutrients and trace minerals, even though my caloric intake was severely reduced. I was pleasantly surprised that I was not hungry. I was in the wonderful world of nutritional abundance, which has nothing to do with calories. The body only cares about nutrients that can be absorbed.

As my body was optimally supplied with the necessary nutrients in minimal calories, it naturally began to detoxify itself by utilizing the massive amounts of these nutrients. I call some of these specific nutrients toxin hunters. **The job of a toxin hunter is to break down toxins so they become water soluble and pass out harmlessly through the liver and the kidneys**.

The essential mineral suites support enzymes that naturally occur in the body. Impurities stored in fat cells traveled to my liver to be detoxified. The liver then released these impurities as bile or converted them into water-soluble waste to be processed by my liver and excreted from my body through the colon. This process differs from a colon cleanse, which is designed to release toxins only in the colon, not the toxins stored in our fat cells.

WHY DOES NUTRITIONAL FASTING PRODUCE SUCH DRAMATIC RESULTS?

During my personal nutritional fasting experience, antioxidant botanicals such as Aloe gel, licorice root, and ashwagandha root supported liver detoxification and reduced my cravings. My body was consistently and sufficiently nourished with nutritious elements and essential ionic macro minerals, micro minerals, and trace elements instead of empty calories.

Even when my body was immersed in a Nutritional Fasting day, I was continually satisfied. For the first time in my life I was fortified with the appropriate amounts of nutrition and mineral suites—a need that extends far beyond just calories. This is a new paradigm in nutritional science. After enlisting in this program, it forever changed my perceptions of the true meaning of health. I now know it is not the number of calories that matter in achieving a healthy lifestyle, but the make-up of nutrition that is contained within those calories. What our bodies really require are nutrient-dense super calories.

The Nutritional Super Calorie

Imagine that a new gasoline additive was invented that allowed cars to get 100 or 200 miles per gallon instead of 20 miles per gallon. The same concept lies behind the nutritional super calorie. Just as the car would use much less gasoline and still travel much farther, this nutritional fasting approach provides the body with significantly more nutrients in fewer calories. The body is able to function much more efficiently on less food.

For me, the nutritional fasting approach extends beyond a weight-loss program. By experiencing these extraordinarily dense foods, and the super-nutritional calories they contain, I was catapulted into a lifestyle where I began to maximize my quality of life potential for the first time in my life. I now have more energy, sharpened mental clarity, and a new zest for life. These benefits are just as significant as the weight loss I achieved. Nutritional fasting set me on a path toward youthful aging, longevity, and a maximization of my life's potential. I've achieved a state of well-being that keeps me energized and engaged constantly in my daily life. It allows me for the first time to achieve two critical goals: first and foremost, to live healthier and longer; and second, to maximize my wellness and human potential. Along with my increased energy and improved mental clarity, I have lower stress and boundless energy. I even sleep like a baby. These are only a few of the benefits I experienced.

I hear countless stories about how people are getting so much more out of nutritional fasting than just the weight loss and the fat they are releasing, and I'll share some of these stories with you in chapter seven.

I received a call from a woman named Sharon, who had been on the nutritional fasting approach for only 6 days of her first 30 days. Sharon said she was amazed at the amount of energy she had and she couldn't believe how well she was sleeping. Although she started the program because she wanted to lose weight, she now says the energy and the deep sleep she gets far surpass the weight she is releasing quickly and safely.

*   *   *

You now have the specifics for how to follow the nutritional fasting program to maximize your wellness potential as well as a better understanding of exactly how it works and why it's so successful. In the next chapter we'll explore how to sustain your momentum, handle any plateaus, and remain motivated.

Chapter Six

Sustaining Your Health Momentum

People ask me all the time, "Do I have to do this for the rest of my life?" My answer is always the same. It starts with a question, and that question is, "Why wouldn't you want to do a little nutritional fasting every day?" Toxins don't go on vacation or mysteriously disappear from our world.

If you do not continue to resupply the body with glutathione (from whey or the vegan shakes) and polysaccharides (from the inner heart gel of Aloe vera) then you will severely reduce the body's natural ability to detoxify itself.

So, I would ask this question instead: "Why wouldn't you want to continue to supply your body on a daily basis with the very molecules that give our bodies the natural ability to detoxify itself?" Toxins simply don't go away once you stop the program. Toxins are entering our bodies 24/7, 365 days a year, and they never take a day off.

MAINTAINING YOUR NEW LIFESTYLE

An important reason to continue drinking these whey protein shakes is that our bodies do not store protein—or the amino acids it imparts. We store fats and carbohydrates, but not protein. Plus, chicken, fish, soy, and many other forms of protein simply don't have the levels of nutrients our bodies need, such as the amino acids and the added ionic minerals and trace elements.

Also, other than breast milk, carefully selected, raw, undenatured whey protein shakes are simply unsurpassed as a source of protein to reduce the risk of sarcopenia (loss of muscle mass) and to supply your body with the nutrients that allows it to continue nutritional fasting. Scientists agree that undenatured whey protein on its own is necessary for optimal health. With the addition of essential minerals and trace elements and enzymes, super shakes should include ingredients that are essential to the human body. It's no wonder we've named them "super" shakes. It should be obvious why consuming a super shake each morning has so many advantages over any other food you can possibly consume.

GLUTATHIONE'S CRITICAL ROLE IN DETOX

In her book *Detoxify or Die*, Sherry Rogers, MD, explains that every time the antioxidant glutathione goes out and hunts and then pulls apart and renders a toxin harmless, the glutathione gives up its life. In other words, **for every molecule of a toxin that glutathione destroys safely, we lose one molecule of glutathione as well.** The same is true for the toxin hunter's polysaccharides. If glutathione and poly-saccharides are doing their job, then we must continually replace and replenish the depleted stocks of both as they continue to detoxify our bodies—every day.

In other words, if you do not continue to resupply the body with glutathione (from whey or vegan shakes) and polysaccharides (from the inner-heart gel of Aloe vera) then you will severely reduce the body's natural ability to detoxify itself.

Marco Ruggiero, MD, who has a PhD in Molecular Biology and is a professor at the University of Florence in experimental oncology, also believes in the importance of whey protein. He is recognized as one of the lead researchers in the world on our immune system. Dr. Ruggiero has published more than 160 scientific papers in major peer-reviewed scientific journals on topics as diverse as the critical role macrophages (the main soldiers of our immune system) play in supporting the immune system. Two of his papers rank in the top 10 percent of all scientific papers ever published.

Simply put, macrophages are large cells in the body capable of enrobing and destroying foreign entities, viruses and free radicals. Macrophages are essentially the first line of defense against invasions of infections and viruses in the body. His paper on macrophages[11] which was published in the prestigious journal *Nutrients*, is in the top 5 percent of all scientific published papers in history up to this time. This is why Dr. Ruggiero is considered one of the world's experts on the role of macrophages and their critical role in supporting the immune system.

He has stated that "the food" for our macrophages is protein. In his clinics in Switzerland, Germany, and England, he uses raw carefully selected, undenatured whey protein with all of his patients, regardless of their severe health challenges. This is the same raw, carefully selected, undenatured whey protein that we recommend as the cornerstone of *TDOS Solutions'* nutritional fasting approach.

Dr. Ruggiero asks these questions:

1. Why wouldn't you want to feed your macrophages one of the best protein sources in the world?

2. Don't you want to maximize the effectiveness of your macrophages?

3. What are you feeding your macrophages today?

As you can see, the TDOS solutions are a lifelong commitment to health. If you want to continue eliminating the dangerous toxins in your body and ensure that you are receiving the right nutrients, then it's critical to continue this program as a way of life.

BOOSTING YOUR TOXIN HUNTERS

Yet another critical toxin hunter that works the same way (for each molecule of toxin, the body uses up one of these other toxin hunters) is called a polysaccharide. It is contained in the inner-heart filet of the Aloe vera plant. Unless you continually assist the body in re-supplying these toxin hunters in large quantities, you will succumb to the toxic armies of the TDOS Syndrome as they attack you every day.

There is no other option for me. I will consume the Super Shake and Super Aloe Vera Mineral Drink each morning of my life, as I choose a nutritional fasting healthy lifestyle that is more than 11 years old and way beyond "my first 30 days."

HANDLING MAINTENANCE AND PLATEAUS

At this point, you may be wondering how to sustain results, maintain long-term weight loss, and, more important, continue to naturally detox. Every day, some level of nutritional fasting is recommended for maintaining weight, natural detoxification, and maximizing your optimal wellness potential. I've accomplished this by consuming two ounces of the aloe vera juice enhanced with the "mineral suites" each morning (the Super Aloe Vera Mineral Drink), along with a raw, carefully selected, undenatured whey protein shake (the Super Shake) to sustain the levels of necessary nutrients, vitamins, and essential minerals needed to maintain my fat-burning processes.

I drink another two ounces of the Aloe vera super juice before going to sleep to continuously assist natural detoxification of my body of everyday toxins and impurities. I also engage in a two-day nutritional fast once every two months to rid my body of those deeply embedded impurities trapped in fat cells.

Though it is important to continue to select from the list of recommended foods on page shown on page 44 and again on page 126 after completing the nutritional fast, it does not mean that "guilty pleasure" foods such as pizza, ice cream, or alcohol cannot be enjoyed in a nutritional fasting lifestyle—as long as they are consumed in moderation. We believe in living your life in moderation. Too much of anything is going to present a problem. With that being said, following a program like this allows people to still enjoy what they want. We would never tell people to follow a program that we don't or can't follow. Once you figure out how this program works with your body, you will know how to find a balance between eating foods you enjoy and splurging on vacations and what it takes when you return home to get back to your ideal health and weight.

After completing the TDOS Solution's nutritional fasting approach, if you begin to experience food cravings again or become fatigued, overwhelmed, or depressed while on the maintenance program, this could be a warning sign that your body has returned to sugar-burning mode. Sugar-burning mode is good for a very short period of time if you are going to run a 100-yard dash, but the body was meant to burn fat for long-term energy. In sugar-burning mode you will constantly seek out sugars and carbs to replace the sugar that is rapidly used up by your body.

Fat burning produces much higher energy and more long-term energy. The sooner you can enter and maintain fat burning, the more energy you will have and the better you will feel. You can combat sugar burning by immediately completing just one nutritional fasting cycle to return your body to detoxifying mode to burn off toxic fat.

As is the case with traditional diets, it is possible to hit a plateau. These plateau periods may indicate that the body has slowed down or stopped detoxifying or that too many simple carbohydrates, refined sugars, or artificial sweeteners have been reintroduced into the diet to cause the body to enter starvation mode from the overconsumption of empty calories. Otherwise, the body may have achieved a state of equilibrium and will retain fluid for a period of time until a new equilibrium point is set, causing the body to dump the excess fluid.

The key during any of these plateau periods is to not get discouraged, and to continue to self-motivate with the prospect of enhanced energy and vibrant wellness of mind, body, and spirit.

A LONG-TERM COMMITMENT THAT YIELDS EXTRAORDINARY RESULTS

The recommendations set forth in the TDOS Solution's approach in this book are designed to help you achieve a nutritional fasting lifestyle. Recognize toxicity as the cause for systemic problems throughout the body and treat the body as a whole to truly solve them. And although single-point solutions are helpful in certain applications, specific-point nutrients cannot deal with the systemic needs to maintain overall wellness of the body.

I have found that the TDOS Solution approach is a major breakthrough in nutritional science and it is "the one." It is the real deal as they say. Never before have so many people had consistent, long-term, life-changing-results day after day, month after month, year after year. This is the first real long-term solution that can lead to a long-term healthy life. The solution formulas are so successful because they include specific nutrients that allow the body to manufacture more of what it is lacking on its own. Anytime the body can make more of what it requires, especially when it comes to detox, it is always more effective. The nutrients in the nutritional formulas we have laid out for you to look for replenish our bodies with the nutrients they require that we cannot obtain in our foods. This is why the TDOS Solutions really do make every calorie count that you consume.

The nutritional fasting healthy lifestyle choice is a step toward reducing our "toxic burdens" and ultimately sets us on the path toward long-term health and wellness. The many other TDOS Solutions co-factors are also critical components in maximizing our quality of life potential and assisting our bodies in remaining healthy.

Those who need to lose weight normally say "my scale must be broken," when they see dramatic weight loss typically occur in a very short period of time.

Those who do the nutritional fast because they like the idea of giving their cells an "oil change" often say "I really did not believe it was possible to feel this good. I have more energy than I have ever had and I just feel wonderful." Athletes are amazed at the improvement in their lean muscle mass, drastic improvements in their athletic performance, and their quick recovery time after working out.

Dr. Ruggiero said "food is the genetic information that we communicate to our genes."

What kind of genetic information are your food choices communicating to your genes?

YOUR OWN PERSONAL SOLUTION ADVISORS

We realize you may still have questions before getting started, based on your own individual goals or maybe you just need more information. If you do need additional information or support, please visit www.theGreenlawReport.com and enlist the help of the Solution Providers at Epic Seasons. They are available to answer any and all of your questions, and they will advise you through the nutritional fast for free. Because each person is different, these advisors can assist you in the best way to start so that you can reach your goal of getting to maintenance as safely and quickly as possible. For people with health challenges, the solution advisors, in many cases, can modify the program accordingly to make it better fit your individual needs. (Solution Advisors are not healthcare professionals and you should always check with your own health professional or doctor before starting this nutritional fasting solution.)

The most important concept I have repeated numerous times is that the real reason to complete the nutritional fast is simple: "to live healthier for as long as you can." I don't know a single human being on this planet who is not interested in that. I leave you to decide.

THE ROLE OF EXERCISE IN NUTRITIONAL FASTING

Once you are familiar with what to expect on each day of a nutritional fasting program, you can introduce exercise into your daily routine. However, we do not recommend starting a nutritional fast and a new exercise program at the same time.

When beginning this program, I was advised to walk at least 30–60 minutes every day, preferably in the morning, to promote fat burning. Though I was told a 60-minute walk was ideal, I was only able to walk for 15 minutes at a time. I walked twice a day for 15 minutes, working up to 30 minutes. When I could, I also jumped on a mini trampoline for 30 minutes.

By combining exercise and nutrient-rich foods, my body functioned efficiently by burning fat for energy. For me, weight loss was a side benefit of my newfound nutritional fasting lifestyle. Adhering to the recommended regimen and consistently ingesting the unique combination of ingredients from my protein shake, I allowed my body to naturally cleanse so I could accomplish long-term optimal health and wellness, extend my longevity, and maximize my potential.

Chapter Seven

Nutritional Fasting Personal Transformations

For me, the Nutritional Fasting approach goes far beyond a weight-loss program. By experiencing these extraordinarily dense foods, and the super-nutritional calories they contain, I was catapulted into a lifestyle of full wellness. I now have more energy, sharpened mental clarity, and a new zest for life. These benefits are as significant as the weight loss I achieved. I hear countless stories about how people are getting so much more out of nutritional fasting than simply the pounds they are releasing.

Even my personal trainer Christian, who is twenty-six years old, recently told me that he cannot believe how this program has helped him reduce his overall body fat percentage, increase his flexibility, and decrease his recovery time after workouts. This is a young man already in incredible shape, and it further enhanced and improved his performance. Although a skeptic at first, Christian now follows the TDOS Solutions and recommends them to his clients. In this chapter, we'll share personal transformations from a few different men and women who've had enormous success on the program.

COACH MIKE MACINTYRE DROPS 68 POUNDS

Consider the amazing story of University of Colorado Head Football Coach, Mike MacIntyre, who lost many pounds quickly—and safely—to transform his life. Mike MacIntyre was introduced to the TDOS

Solutions one winter, and by the dog days of the next summer, Mac-Intyre was back to his high school weight! He shared his story with us for this book.

"I had just wrapped up my first season coaching in Colorado and was visiting family in Nashville. I woke up late one night on that vacation and had this epiphany. I looked into the mirror and didn't recognize the man staring back at me. Like most people, my weight gain was slow but consistent. It's not like I woke up one morning 60 pounds overweight, but it wasn't until that night in Nashville when I really noticed that I had to make some changes. On that same trip, I saw my doctor and he confirmed that change was necessary. As an athlete my entire life, I was in foreign territory as far as what to do to get healthy. I knew I couldn't continue on the path I was traveling, but did I need to diet or work out? I was filled with questions and concerns."

Coach MacIntyre returned to Colorado determined to make the necessary changes to lead a healthy life. Just a few days after having his "aha" moment, Mike attended a sports banquet and, by chance, had a conversation with Peter Greenlaw.

"I remember listening to Peter speak, and his story resonated with me. What he shared with me was thought provoking and it made a lot of sense. Yes, there were a few things I knew I was doing that weren't the best for optimal living, but I also did not know how I had gotten to this point. My diet had not drastically changed over the past several years, and my lifestyle had stayed consistent, so where did this extra weight come from? I knew after meeting Peter that I was supposed to be in that room to hear what he shared with me, and I thought, maybe this was the way I could start to help myself. Peter gave me his first book, *Why Diets Are Failing Us*. I read it and decided to give it a shot. I was still a bit skeptical when I started, but I was desperate for a change and hoped this would be the catalyst."

On January 1, 2014, Coach MacIntyre started on the solution. With some general help from a Solution Advisor, he was on his way to recapturing a healthy lifestyle. It took him just 11 days to see a drastic change in his health and his waistline.

MacIntyre's timing on changing his health coincided with one of his busiest times of the year: recruiting season. Most weeks saw MacIntyre traveling the country and visiting with future players and their families. Because of this, he had to make sure the TDOS Solution was flexible enough for him to make time for meals with the families he visited.

"When traveling, and visiting with kids, it's not uncommon to meet them over a meal. I could not just walk into these homes and not eat with the family—or turn down some amazing home cooking from around the country! Fortunately, I was able to work with a Solution Advisor and come up with a customized plan to keep me on track, while still enjoying the company and food on the recruiting trail."

In roughly a few months, MacIntyre lost 68 pounds, and he has dramatically changed his eating habits. He completely eliminated diet soda and now drinks mostly water. Instead of feeling like he needs caffeine all the time, he keeps water with him. He's now also able to get back into the gym.

Mike and his family were not the only ones to notice his dramatic health change since the end of last football season. As spring and summer practices fired up for the upcoming season, so did the press and interviews surrounding Coach MacIntyre and his team.

"I would be in a press conference regarding the team's progress, and I would get all these questions regarding my weight loss and health and how I did it! A couple articles were published on my new approach on health. It has been a great confidence booster for me. I know my players really respect what I have done, and I now use my story to help motivate them."

In just a few weeks, we have seen people lose tremendous amounts of weight that would take months with conventional diets. This, of course, gives them a reason to believe this new solution is the real answer to long-term weight loss, maximizing their wellness potential and the real road to living healthier longer. Once they are able to get to the simple TDOS Solutions maintenance plan, they realize that the weight is not coming back.

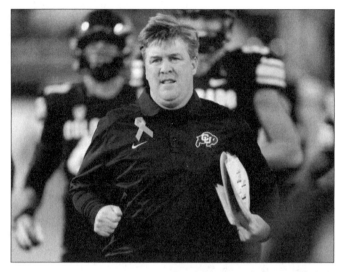

Coach MacIntyre before weight loss

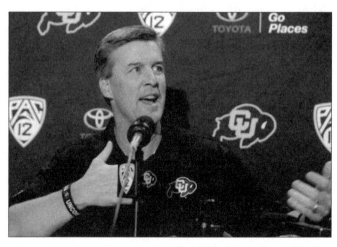

Coach MacIntyre after weight loss

MIKE TOWNSEND LOSES 170 POUNDS . . . SAFELY

As Mike stated to me, describing why he took the step to change the direction of his life, "I made the decision to recapture my health." Looking back, Mike Townsend may not have even realized at the time that a phone call to get some information on a nutritional fasting program would propel him into a rebirth—and a second chance at a healthy life.

We first met Mike several years ago when he was desperate for a change. After trying countless programs promising extreme weight loss by using everything from diet pills to support groups. Nothing had ever worked for him and he came to us as skeptic as anyone. He had literally tried everything on the market and had seen little to no results. Reluctantly, he agreed to try the program for a week.

"Just the week before," said Mike, "I had spent several hundred dollars on a weight-loss program, which I had already returned. In fact, when this new package showed up, I called the number I was given to see how I could return the stuff, as I already knew it wouldn't work. The lady who answered that call gave me just enough inspiration to try it and, ultimately, it helped change my life."

The lady Mike spoke with was one of our Solution Advisors, and she convinced him to get through the first four days before making his final decision. Those four days made enough of an impression that, three years later, he has completely changed his lifestyle.

These days, you won't catch Mike flipping through television reruns. In fact, you might not catch him at all, as he averages between 20- to 30-mile bike rides each day, when the weather cooperates. Since May of 2012, he has ridden more than 5,500 miles on his road bike. Three years ago, the idea of getting on a bike would not have crossed his mind. Not only is Mike an avid bike rider but also he found a second home at the gym, working with a personal trainer, and has completely switched his dietary needs. In less than a year's time, he lost 170 pounds. Even more important, after three years, he has managed to keep off the weight.

Mike offers insight to others who want to take a similar path: "Every day is still a battle. I still deal with a fat man's mentality. I don't know if I will ever be the person who can eat just one. Three years into this program and I still slip. I will do really well for seven or eight weeks and then have a week where I want to eat everything in sight. Luckily, I know how to regain control now. I have also learned so much through this experience that guilt plays a positive role where I can use it to launch me out of a funk and back on track. For me, one of the biggest elements of this program is that I still can enjoy food in moderation. And, if I get sidetracked, I know what I need to do to get right back to where I want."

"For years, I was stuck in my own deception. I would look in the mirror and not see the person who was really staring back at me. I didn't become majorly overweight overnight. Every year, I would put on 10-15 pounds. When it happens like that, you don't notice how big you are really getting until 20 years down the line. I also knew that going into this program, I wasn't going to lose all that excess weight quickly. All the other programs I had tried just did not satisfy me, results wise. It was hard to cut calories and meals or work my butt off in the gym to lose a pound here and there. After just a couple weeks on this solution, I had lost a double-digit percentage of weight! I was so excited that I forgot how it was actually working; I just kept doing it!"

After six months on the program, Mike Townsend has never looked back. He lost almost a pound a day for that first six months. Because of his dramatic weight loss, Mike now faced a new problem: purchasing a new wardrobe. He went from a size 54-inch waist to a 34! Today, he still fits happily in his 34-inch jeans.

Mike went from eating two, foot-long sub sandwiches, a family-size bag of chips, and a 64-ounce soda for lunch, to blending up a nutrient-dense protein shake and noticing the same satisfaction. To say he has changed his lifestyle is an understatement. Mike is also proof that this solution is not a one-hit wonder. After the course of

Mike Townsend's Before and After Gallery

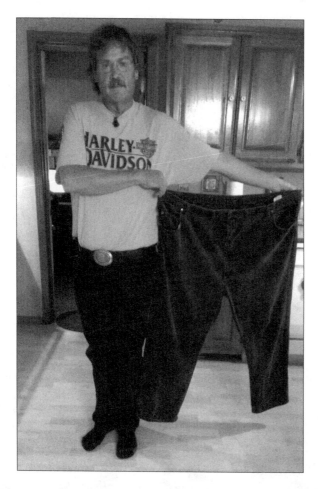

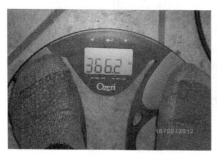
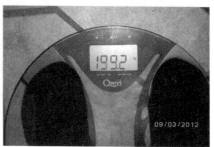

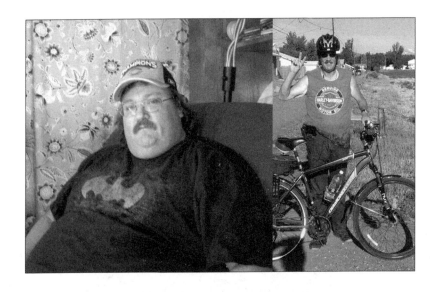

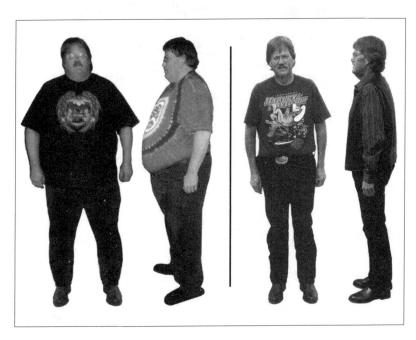

three years, with all the trials and tribulations that life throws at someone, he is living proof that following the guidelines laid out in this book really does work.

Mike also stresses the importance of working with a Solution Advisor. She played the roles of educator, motivator, cheerleader, and sometimes butt kicker in Mike's case. "The fact that there was someone out there that wanted to help me and was concerned about my well-being meant a lot to me," he said.

One of the ways that Mike stayed accountable to himself was by becoming a solution advisor himself.

Helping others is really what keeps Mike going. "I owe it to the newcomer to keep going. I want to be the inspiration to that guy who was like me three years ago. You never know who you may help out there and that's what I am all about."

Mike has lived the story that some of us may never have to. With that story comes great power. He has a realistic approach to working with people that is the definition of genuine. Over the past three years, Mike has proven that the techniques laid out in this book really do work. He has seen a dramatic physical transformation, and equally as important, a mental one. He is one of our favorite success stories and has become one of the most beloved advisors. "The best way I can help is by sharing my story and by practicing what I preach."

JILL FULFILLS A LIFELONG DREAM

Jill came to us after countless failed attempts from a myriad of programs and was ready for more of the same. The fact that this seemed different than all the standard calorie counting programs out there was the one reason she agreed to give it a shot.

"In the 3rd grade, my school nurse put me on the scale. She proceeded to tell me that I was fat and weighed more than she did. In that moment, at the tender age of eight, for the first time I became ashamed of my weight. This single moment in time became a major catalyst in shaping my entire life and sparked a lifetime of struggle with my health, weight, and body image."

"Fast forward 30 years, another singular moment locked in time when I was swimming with my family. My kids begged me to go down the pool slide. Before I knew it, I was wedged within the slide. As minutes passed, a family member worked on getting me out. Finally, out I came, mortified."

"Through the years, I tried literally everything to lose weight. I took my 'before' pictures 24 times, each time saying to myself, 'this time I'll do it.' I failed every time, which only worsened my weight battle and food addictions."

"In April of 2010, I hit my bottom. I was desperate to break the vicious circle that had imprisoned me for the majority of my life. I even tried out for *The Biggest Loser.* I made it to the semi-finals, however I wasn't selected to appear on the show. I promised my close friend that if I wasn't selected, I would try this new approach of nutritional fasting. With faith that God would help me conquer my addictions, I made good on my promise."

"My journey began the same time the Biggest Loser contestants went to the ranch to start on their journey. I made a vision board with the 100 Pound Club as my main goal. I eased into a light exercise program and religiously followed my new nutritional protocol. I was finally driven!"

"When *The Biggest Loser* finale aired, my personal results actually surpassed all the female contestants as I had achieved a higher percentage of weight loss than any other woman on the show! Overall, I released 131 pounds (half my body weight) and have gone from a size 22 to a size four, which I also had written on my vision board!"

"My new body has allowed me to accomplish things I never thought possible. For example, my son and I recently climbed to the top of a mountain near St. George. As we sat side by side on the summit,

Jill's Before and After photos

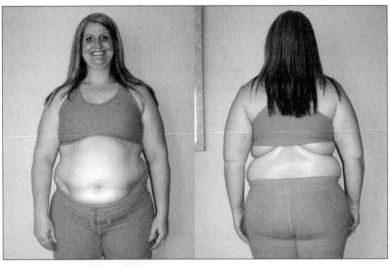

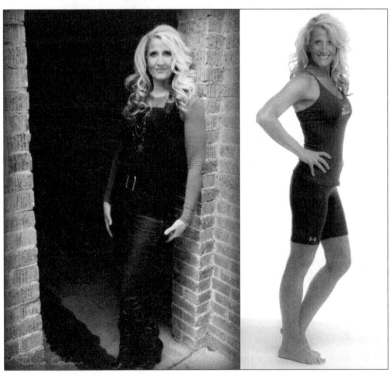

he turned to me with tears in his eyes and said, 'Mom, you did it! Thanks for getting healthy for us!' Just a year earlier, my son had been embarrassed when I came to his school because someone told him he had a fat mom. I recently completed three half-marathons, yet another goal on my vision board!"

"With these priceless moments, I've realized that I will never again sit on the sidelines. I am now capable of living life to the fullest, achieving new milestones, creating new memories with loved ones, and expecting the unexpected!"

"I believe everyone should feel as exuberant as I do today. There were times when I doubted I would ever achieve the health goals I set out to reach, and it was a process, but the rewards are infinite. I've gained self-confidence and feel as though I have a new lease on life. In return, I'm fortunate to currently be helping thousands of people become the person God intended them to be. I know people can change their destiny as I did and it is so rewarding to give back and help these people realize their dreams can come true just like they did for me!"

* * *

Hopefully these stories have encouraged you to remain on the TDOS Solutions program, with the knowledge that you can lose weight quickly and safely while simultaneously detoxifying your body. You are also likely enjoying the added benefits of having more energy, improved athletic performance, and achieving your own personal goals. In part III we'll provide the specific ingredients and recipes you'll need to succeed as we'll as some additional information on the reasons behind why protein and amino acids are so critical to your health.

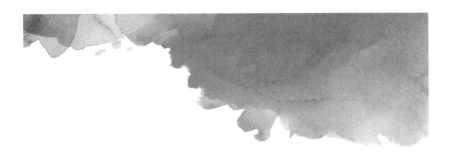

PART THREE

The TDOS Solutions
Nutritional Fast

Chapter Eight

How to Create Your TDOS Solutions: The Critical Ingredients

Now that you know how to follow the program and have read about alternating Super Shake Days with Deep Nutritional Fasting Days and Feast Days in chapter five, this chapter will provide you with more specific information about the ingredients your shakes should and should not contain as well as the recipes for making these powerful drinks on your own.

SUPER SHAKES: SUPER WHEY

Raw, Carefully Selected, Undenatured Whey Protein Shake

This formula will allow you to create an extraordinary whey shake, built on a superior protein base and fortified with some of our friends from the Mineral Suites. There two important parts to this shake— both what it contains, and what it does not contain.

Following are the necessary ingredients you need from a fulfillment company of your choice:

- **Raw Whey Protein**—carefully selected, undenatured whey protein from grass-fed cows that are not injected with antibiotics or growth hormones. It is suggested the minimum target protein quantity per shake should be 24 grams with a high preferred amino acid profile.

- **Proteases**–enzymes that help to break down protein into particles called peptides that makes the amino acids much easier to be utilized by the human body

- **Lactase Enzymes**–this can further reduce lactose for those who are lactose intolerant

- **Lipase Enzymes**–Helps to break down fat and works synergistically with lactase to enhance your shake's effectiveness

- **Prebiotic Fiber**–from a mix of flax seed and Iso-maltooligosaccharides to help regulate glucose (if you use natural sweeteners) and enhance good gut bacteria, essential for immune health

- **The Mineral Suites**–this is what we call the essential major minerals (macro minerals), micro minerals (trace minerals), and essential trace elements (see chapter two for a complete list)

- **Good Fats**–olive, sunflower, or coconut oil

- **Vitamin D and Oleic Acid**–from olive oil, these have been shown to add tremendous support for the immune system

Optionally, molasses or stevia can be used as a sweetener if you need one. Stevia contains no sugar and is naturally derived from the stevia plant. Just be sure to read labels carefully as some items claiming to be stevia actually contain added chemicals. There are some clever marketing ploys out there, so be sure to check ingredients on look-alike products like "Truvia," whose primary ingredient isn't stevia at all, but a sugar alcohol called erythritol. Also, stevia is much sweeter than sugar, so use in moderation. As a result, these shakes can taste great, yet they still have a low glycemic index.

Your Shakes Should NOT Contain:

1. Artificial flavorings

2. Artificial sweeteners

3. Soy or soy-derived ingredients

4. Genetically modified organism (GMO) ingredients

5. Gluten or wheat

When you make your super shake daily with the additional nutritionally dense ingredients, you will feel really satisfied because of the massive number of nutrients contained within each shake. Remember, the key to satisfying our hunger is nutritional density, not how many calories we eat. This food is the genetic information we communicate to our genes. This is why it is so critical to make every calorie count.

AN IMPORTANT NOTE: Many shakes on the market today only contain 8 to 10 grams of protein, which experts say is woefully short of what the body needs to maximize its wellness potential. Additionally, many advertised shakes contain only 90 to 110 calories and lack many of the properties and/or the nutrients in raw, carefully selected, undenatured whey protein shakes. The end result is that you end up hungry in an hour or so, no matter what the slick ads promise.

SUPER SHAKES: SUPER VEGAN

For people who are vegan or lactose intolerant, a substitute vegan shake can be used. The challenge with vegan shakes is that they must contain combined proteins from several different plant proteins to be effective. For example, a vegan shake based solely on pea protein is insufficient to do the heavy lifting in assisting the body in removing toxins. The reason a single source of vegetable protein by itself is not an effective toxin hunter is that it does not have a high enough amino acid profile.

To use a vegan shake as an effective weapon against toxicity, it must contain several sources of vegetable proteins combined in one shake. When careful attention is paid to the nutritional profile, a vegan shake can be highly effective in creating a preventive intervention to toxins and to living healthier longer.

Raw, carefully selected, undenatured whey protein is generally regarded the world over as a great source for high levels of amino acids. The great news is that by combining several vegetable proteins, you can achieve almost the same amino acid profile as whey protein. We recommend a shake that contains at least 24 grams of protein derived from a blend of pea and whole brown rice proteins. When combined, these can provide a complete amino acid profile similar to that of whey protein shakes.

If you add a few more ingredients, your heart and blood vessels will thank you. You'll want to include healthy fats from sources including extra virgin olive oil and sunflower oil (monounsaturated fats), flax and chia seed (omega-3s, -6s, and -9s), and coconut-derived medium-chain triglycerides. And, your belly will benefit from dietary fiber that includes a mix of chia seed and gut-healthy prebiotics like inulin and oligosaccharides.

QUICK REFERENCE FOR OPTIMAL
VEGAN SHAKE INGREDIENTS

Use combined proteins from several different plants with a high amino-acid profile and extra virgin olive oil or sunflower oil (or another monounsaturated fat), flax and chia seeds, omega-3, omega-6, and omega-9 fatty acids, coconut-derived medium-chain triglycerides, inulin, oligosaccharides, mineral suites, vitamin D-3, and Oleic Acid.

Additional Micronutrients Needed

This vegetarian meal alternative also should possess its own "whole foods" base of micronutrients (to retain vitamins and phytochemicals) and juice powders from natural foods. These should include a variety of fruits, vegetables (carrots and beets), and nuts.

Sprouts, vegetables, and fruits are the sources for naturally occurring vitamins. It is also important that these fruits, sprouts, and vegetables be carefully processed by using a low temperature, spray-drying process, which preserves the natural ingredients. This will ensure that these are unprocessed foods containing all their natural vitamins and phytochemicals. If a process other than low temperature spray drying is used, the specific vitamins and phytochemicals can be greatly diminished or totally destroyed. That is why there is such an importance placed on how foods are processed. Once you understand that we need nutrients in their natural state after processing, you will understand that processing is as important as their nutritional density.

Your vegan shake must also not contain any artificial colors, ingredients from genetically modified organisms (GMOs), or any soy ingredients.

Healthy Fats and Fiber

In addition to the vegan protein combinations, sprouts, and vitamins, you need a few more components. There is convincing evidence that we also require healthy fats, carbohydrates, and dietary fiber.

Consider these healthy fats just like in the whey protein shake: a mix of sunflower oil, extra virgin olive oil, flax, coconut—offering monounsaturated and polyunsaturated fats (omega-3s, omega-6s, omega-9) as well as medium-chain triglycerides. Be careful, as most other vegan shakes on the market only supply soy oil comprised of mainly omega-6s.

As previously stated, a great dietary fiber should include prebiotic soluble oligosaccharides and inulin to promote growth of good bacteria in the digestive tract. This prebiotic fiber is so important because periodic fiber (not probiotic fiber) is the preferred fuel source for the primary good bacteria in the gut and this, in turn, can help reduce the growth of bad bacteria.

In addition, the perfect vegan shake includes insoluble fiber from flax and chia seed for bulk and regularity.

Vegan Shakes Not Just for Vegetarians

There are a record number of people with sensitivities to different foods, such as dairy, soy, or eggs. Vegan shakes offer a fantastic alternative, not just for those who avoid animal products entirely, but for those with lactose intolerance or a milk allergy.

Our ancestral past as hunters and gatherers, suggests that we should incorporate a wide variety of foods, including nuts, berries, fruits, and vegetables into our diets. This is because there are vital micronutrients in these whole foods—micronutrients that we need to maintain healthy bodies and support all the building blocks we need.

Remember, your body is completely capable of detoxifying itself. This naturally occurs through caloric reduction and intermittent nutritional fasting. It is important that you have massive amounts of nutrients in the reduced calories. This is a critical difference between the TDOS Solutions doctor-recommended approach and conventional diets, which rely exclusively on lowering calories without a corresponding increase in nutrients per calories. Without the increased nutrients, you will go into metabolic shutdown and starvation mode, which causes the body to store fat and burn muscle.

This is why on a conventional diet doctors warn patients not to lose more than a pound a week. They're right—if you are on a conventional diet, you don't want to lose more than a pound a week, because you typically lose lean muscle mass.

Fortunately, the TDOS Solution's caloric reduction (not nutrient reduction) and nutritional fasting is not a diet. It does not put the body into starvation mode, and thus drastically reduces the risk of losing lean muscle mass. Best of all, the TDOS Solution produces results in a matter of days—not weeks—safely.

THE DETOX DRINK

Super Aloe Vera Mineral Drink

In order for you to select the best mineral drink for supporting your body as it detoxes, combine Aloe vera inner heart gel and the essential mineral suites. Don't forget—it's your body doing the work here.

This unique formulation (recipe) you choose must contain aloe vera gel made from the inner-heart filet of the Aloe vera plant that has been processed at low temperatures and spray-dried to preserve the enzymes and nutrients.

The inner-heart filet is where the Aloe plant stores the majority of its nutrients, enzymes, essential amino acids, vitamins, and minerals—all of which support digestive health and the immune system, while assisting the body in detoxification.

This inner-filet of the Aloe plant also contains polysaccharides (which we call natural toxin hunters), substances that have been touted for their ability to balance the immune system, work as natural detoxifiers, and encourage the liver's biochemical, toxin-neutralizing processes. The polysaccharides simply support the body in the natural detox process, which it is capable of carrying out if it has the right assistance. We call polysaccharides natural toxin hunters because their job is to go out and break toxins apart, rendering them water soluble. They can then pass through the kidneys and liver safely and easily.

To top it all off, make sure this drink includes the essential mineral suites outlined in Chapter Two. These nutritionally-dense ingredients treat the body to relieve it of excess and nutritionally bankrupt waste. The body can then perform the way it was intended and self-regulate to achieve optimal health, maximize potential, and live healthier longer.

NOT ALL ALOE VERA IS CREATED EQUALLY

Use caution when selecting aloe vera. Many Aloe vera supplements use high heat processing that actually destroys the polysaccharides and other nutrients. If a product says "whole leaf Aloe vera," do not use it. Whole leaf Aloe actually contains an enzyme in the leaf that destroys polysaccharides.

Only the inner-heart filet of the *Aloe* plant should be used, and it must be prepared by a low-heat, spray-dried process.

TAKE A SUPER VITAMIN COMBINATION OF BOTANICALS AND CLEANSING HERBS

The human body creates optimal wellness through caloric reduction (not nutritional reduction) and intermittent nutritional fasting to cleanse itself (not colon cleansing) naturally. In order for nutritional fasting to occur, the body must have a massive supply of nutrients but limited calories. The use of a super multivitamin (concentrating on nutritional density) is essential to allow the body to perform its effective ability to rid itself of harmful toxins.

You will want to use a super combination of vitamins, botanicals, cleansing herbs, and essential mineral suites not only to assist the body in natural nutritional fasting but also to combat the devastating effects of nutritional deficiency.

CONSUME PLENTY OF FILTERED WATER

Another overlooked nutrient is filtered water. Yes, filtered water. The human body consists of 70 percent water, the brain is 80 percent water, and the blood is 90 percent water. No other beverage, be it milk, juice, coffee, tea, or soda, can quench the thirst of our cells. Only clean filtered water can do that. Everything else simultaneously hydrates and dehydrates—why else do you think soda has added salt and sugar?

According to Dr. Feredoon Batamanghelidj, regarded as one of the world's experts on water and its impact on the human body, we should all be drinking half our body weight in ounces of water each and every day for optimal health. Anything less than that deprives the cells of the minimum water necessary for proper cell function.

This is a very simple part of the TDOS Solution. This means that if you weigh 160 pounds, you should drink a minimum of 80 ounces of water every day.

TDOS Solutions Guide
for Preparation of Meals and Recipes

Quick Start and Grocery List and Much More!

STEP 1
GETTING STARTED: CLEAN YOUR PANTRY

The following foods and beverages are NOT recommended and should be avoided:

Alcohol, artificial colorings and flavorings, artificial sweeteners, white bread, chips and crackers, cold cuts (unless nitrate-free,) coffee (except for Isagenix low-acid coffee), fresh fruit or dried veggie burgers

Cooking oils that are safflower, sunflower, corn, canola, or peanut oil), deep-fried foods, "enriched foods"

Enriched pasta, excessive salt, fast-food, fruit juice, high-fat cheese, bananas

Instant, packaged foods (like lean cuisine or instant oatmeal), margarine, artificial preservatives

Processed food, refined carbohydrates, shortening products, soda drinks, soy proteins, sugar (including brown sugar, and powdered sugar)

STEP 2
PLAN AHEAD FOR SNACKS AND MEALS

Each snack is designed to tide you over to your next meal and geared toward stabilizing blood sugars. Snacks are NOT meant to fill you up.

Total snacks should contain no more than 300 calories per day. (should be from protein, veggies, or healthy fat)

SNACK SUGGESTIONS

Raw, unsalted almonds, pine nuts, walnuts, brazil nuts. Limit to 4 or 5 nuts. Be sure not to exceed 12 nuts in any 24-hour period.

Organic celery, raw veggies, small green salad, organic hard-boiled eggs

Turkey rolled up in lettuce with veggies, 1/8 of avocado

Organic almond butter or peanut butter on celery or 2 slices of green apple (two teaspoons)

Organic hummus and veggies (1 tablespoon hummus)

Organic guacamole and veggies (1 tablespoon guacamole)

Green tea and mineral-infused chocolates . These are a wonderful chocolates, filled with amino acids that help overcome cravings and balance brain chemistry. They come in dark, dark chocolate mint, milk chocolate, salted caramel, or milk chocolate.

Slimcake (contains gluten)

1 scoop of New Zealand protein with powdered greens

½ serving of New Zealand super shake meal replacement

⅓ meal bar

1–2 oz any lean protein

Choices for Healthy Proteins and Carbs and Good Fats

PROTEIN	GOOD FATS	Fiber-based CARBS
Salmon	Avocado	Romaine Lettuce
Whey Protein (Un-denatured)	Pine Nuts (Raw)	Bell Peppers (All)
Crab/Oysters	Flax Seeds	Green Beans
Tuna	Almonds (Raw)	Celery
Shrimp/Lobster	Walnuts (Raw)	Snow Peas
Halibut	Pecans (Raw)	Zucchini
Canned Sardines	Brazil Nuts (Raw)	Cabbage
Chicken Breast	Tahini	Cucumbers
Lean Beef (95% Fat Free, Grass-Fed and Hormone Free)	Macadamia (Raw)	Broccoli
White Turkey	Avocado Oil (Extra Virgin Cold Pressed)	Artichoke Hearts
Ground Turkey (99% Fat Free)	Almond Butter (Raw Organic)	Asparagus
Rainbow Trout	Coconut Oil Extra Virgin Unrefined Organic)	Cauliflower
Scallops	Almond Oil (Extra Virgin Unrefined Organic)	Endive
Omega 3 Eggs	Raw Butter	Bok Choy

Meal Suggestions

Basic Meal Assembly for Protein Plus Healthy Fat and Veggies and Healthy Oils for Cooking and Eating

CREATING A SALAD

Choose TYPE of Greens (2 to 3 cups)

1. Spinach
2. Broccoli Slaw
3. Mixed Greens
4. Kale Mix

Add ½ to 1 cup vegetables from above

Add 3 oz or 6 oz protein

Add Optional Grain on the side

Dressing: Drizzle to add 1 tablespoon of dressing such as Bragg's Liquid Aminos or Bragg's Sesame Ginger Dressing or organic extra virgin olive oil with lemon and celtic sea salt

SAMPLE LUNCH RECIPES

■ Bowl, wrap, or open-face sandwich

1 serving of grain (brown rice, Ezekiel bread, sprouted tortilla)

3 or 6 oz protein

One cup vegetables of choice

■ Hearty Soup

1 to 2 cups low sodium vegetable broth or chicken broth (organic)

3 to 6 oz of protein

1 cup non-starchy veggies (roasted, grilled or steamed)

½ cup brown rice or brown rice pasta

SAMPLE SMALL MEAL RECIPES

(Breakfast shake, mini-meal, dessert shake)

- ## Zucchini and Sweet Potato Frittata   (Serves 4)

Ingredients

2 tbsp coconut oil or EVOO (olive oil);

8 eggs

1 large sweet potato, peeled and cut in slices

2 sliced zucchinis

1 sliced red bell pepper

2 tbsp fresh parsley

Salt and pepper to taste

Directions

1. Heat a pan over a medium-low heat.

2. Add the oil and sweet potato slices and cook until soft, about 8 minutes.

3. Add the zucchini and red bell pepper slices and cook for another 4 minutes.

4. While it cooks, whisk the eggs in a bowl, making sure to incorporate a lot of air in the mixture.

5. Season the egg mixture with salt and pepper and add to the cooking veggies.

6. Cook on low heat until just set, about 10 minutes.

7. Finish the frittata until golden under a heated broiler.

8. Cut the finished frittata into wedges and serve with fresh parsley.

■ Custom Chicken Packs (You can make a 6 oz portion and split it)

Ingredients

3 oz chicken breast
(can substitute 3 oz salmon, tilapia, or other meaty fish)

*¼ cup organic broccoli florets

1 tsp olive oil (optional) salt and pepper to taste

¼ cup organic salsa
(no sugar added, Green Mountain Gringo Salsa)

*(You can put in any veggie: spinach, asparagus, green beans, etc.)

Directions

1. Preheat oven to 450°F. Combine broccoli, salsa and dressing in medium bowl.

2. For each packet, lay two 20 × 12-inch sheets of regular parchment paper on top of each other.

3. Place 1 chicken breast on each foil packet. Spoon broccoli and salsa mixture equally over each chicken breast. Bring up short sides of each foil packet and double fold top. Double fold both ends to seal each packet, leaving space for steam to gather.

4. Place packets on baking sheet; bake 20 to 25 minutes or until chicken is no longer pink in centers (165°F). Carefully open ends of packets to allow steam to escape before fully opening.

■ Power Chicken Hummus Bowl

3 oz chicken (Applegate makes an organic pre-cooked chicken)

2 to 3 cups spinach with mixed greens

2 T hummus

1/2 cucumber diced

Mix together and enjoy. May add 1/2 cup brown rice or quinoa for starch/grain (for lunch).

■ Stuffed Zucchini Recipe with Brown Rice, Ground Turkey, Red Pepper, and Basil

(Makes 4 servings)

Lunch meal (because it has grain)

2 large or 4 small round zucchini (or use regular shaped zucchini)

½ onion, chopped

½ red bell pepper, chopped ¼

2 tsp. olive oil

1 lb. very lean ground organic turkey/bison/or grass-fed beef

1 tsp. Trader Joe's 21 Spice Seasoning

1 tsp. chopped garlic or garlic puree (from a jar)

½ tsp. ground fennel seed

1 cup cooked brown rice

½ cup finely chopped fresh basil

¼ cup coarsely grated organic parmesan cheese

¼ cup chicken stock

Directions

Preheat oven to 375° F. Cut stem and flower ends off zucchini, trimming off the smallest possible amount of the skin and taking care to cut it off evenly, since this will show. Cut zucchini in half lengthwise.

Then using a pointed teaspoon or melon baller, scoop out and discard most of the zucchini flesh and seeds, leaving an even ½ inch of flesh attached to the skin. If your zucchini are rolling around a lot, you can cut a thin slice on the bottom side of each to make them sit up. Microwave zucchini 3–4 minutes on high.

Heat olive oil in heavy frying pan and sauté chopped onions and peppers until they are soft—about 5 minutes. Remove onions and peppers to large mixing bowl, and then add ground protein to hot pan and cook until starting to brown. When meat is about half cooked, season with the TJ Seasoning and ground fennel. Add garlic, and continue to cook until meat is well browned. Remove cooked protein to mixing bowl.

Add cooked brown rice, chopped basil, parmesan cheese, and chicken stock to protein and vegetable mixture, and gently combine.

Choose a roasting pan with low sides, just big enough to hold the zucchini. Spray pan with nonstick spray or a light misting of olive oil. Stuff zucchini with stuffing mixture, packing in as much as you can into each zucchini, and mounding it up as high as you can, until all stuffing is used.

Put zucchini into roasting pan, putting them close together so they hold each other with stuffing-side up. Roast uncovered 20 to 30 minutes until zucchini is tender-crisp and filling is hot and slightly browned. Serve hot.

This will keep well for a few days in the refrigerator and can be reheated in the microwave.

Recipes for Larger Meals

(Good for Shake, Meal, Shake Days)

■ **Greek Chicken with Roasted Tomatoes**   (6 servings)

You can use leftovers for salads or meals later in week .

Marinade

2 tablespoons Greek seasoning

1 tablespoon lemon zest

1 tablespoon dried oregano

1 teaspoon kosher salt

1 teaspoon black pepper

2 tablespoons olive oil

6 (6 oz) boneless, skinless chicken breasts

2 lbs Roma tomatoes, halved

2 tablespoons extra virgin olive oil

2 tablespoons chopped fresh basil

2 teaspoons minced garlic

1 teaspoon kosher salt

1 teaspoon black pepper

Directions

Combine Greek seasoning, zest, oregano, salt, pepper, oil and chicken in a large zip top bag. Refrigerate overnight. Preheat oven to 400° F. Place chicken on a rimmed baking sheet.

Bake for 25 to 30 minutes or until done.

Place tomatoes, cut side up on a baking sheet. Drizzle with oil, basil, and garlic.

Bake at 400° F for 1 hour, or until browned and soft. Sprinkle with salt and pepper.

■ Herbed Salmon Burgers with Broccoli Slaw   (5 servings)

Ingredients for Salmon Burgers

4 (5 oz) cans boneless, skinless salmon (wild)

2 large eggs or 4 egg whites, lightly beaten

lightly beaten ¼ cup almond flour (Bob's Red Mill, gluten free)

3 tablespoons chopped fresh parsley

2 tablespoons chopped fresh basil

1 small red bell pepper minced

2 teaspoons minced garlic

1 teaspoon kosher salt

1 teaspoon pepper

1 teaspoon olive oil

Ingredients for Broccoli Slaw

¼ cup olive oil

¼ cup apple cider vinegar

1 teaspoon ground mustard

½ teaspoon kosher salt

¼ teaspoon pepper

12 oz organic broccoli slaw mix

Directions for Salmon Burgers

Preheat oven to 375° degrees F.

Wash and drain salmon in a colander. Remove salmon from colander and place in a large bowl with eggs, flour, parsley, basil, bell pepper, garlic, salt and pepper.

Shape mixture into 6 equal patties.

Transfer to a baking sheet lightly covered with olive oil.

Bake for 15 to 18 minutes, or until cooked through.

Directions for Broccoli Slaw

Whisk together oil, vinegar, mustard, salt and pepper in a large bowl. Add slaw mix, and toss to coat. Let stand at least 30 minutes before serving.

■ **Tuna Cakes**   (Servings: 8)

When the drive-through value meal is not an option for you (your standards are way too high for that!), here's a quick and cost-effective meal that delivers both in taste and nutrition. Serve with some plain Greek yogurt mixed with lemon juice and fresh chopped dill.

3 (5oz) cans albacore tuna, in water

2 omega-3 eggs

1 teaspoon lemon juice

2 teaspoons Dijon mustard

2 Tablespoons flax seeds, ground

1 Tablespoon fresh dill, minced; or 1 teaspoon dried dill

dash black pepper

2 Tablespoons olive oil

Directions

Drain the tuna and flake into a medium size bowl. Add the eggs, lemon, Dijon, flax, dill and pepper. Mix well.

In a large skillet place the olive oil over medium heat. Form the tuna mixture into 8 patties. Flatten each patty onto the skillet and cook for 3 minutes per side.

(Nutritional Analysis: 108 calories, 5g fat, 182mg sodium, .4g carbs, .3g fiber, 15g protein)

Dining Out

Keep in mind:
If you are breaking your meals, 2 to 3 oz of chicken is roughly a deck of cards, and 3 oz of fish is the size of a checkbook.

CASUAL DINING

- **Panera Hidden Menu Items:**

1. Power Chicken Hummus Bowl
2. Salmon Caesar (no dressing or croutons)
3. Any salad with protein (no dressing except EVOO and lemon)

- **Chipotle Choices:**

1. Burrito Bowl with chicken, brown rice, lettuce, salsa, fajita veggies
    30g = about 1oz of protein; 120g of protein = 4oz protein
2. Salad with chicken, fajita veggies, lettuce, salsa, dash of cheese
    (see www.chipotle.com You can build your meal—includes calories)

- **Greek Meal in Diner or Deli:**

1. 1 Egg + 2 white scramble or omelette plus
    - a. veggies
    - b. lean protein (chicken sausage)
    - c. salsa
    - d. side of sliced tomatoes
2. Greek Salad with chicken plus
    - a. cucumber slices
    - b. sprinkle of feta (ok) 1/8 cup
    - c. olives
    - d. dressing of olive oil with lemon

3. Kebobs
    a. vegetable
    b. chicken
    c. shrimp
    d. fish

no pita or rice

FINE DINING TIPS

---

1. Return the bread basket. (You won't offend them.)

2. Look for items that say grilled or broiled and ask for no or little oil (you never know what type of oil they use).

3. Order a salad and add protein.

4. Ask for a "doggie bag," and wrap half (if breaking meal into 2 meals).

5. Stick with mainly protein dishes with grilled or roasted vegetables.

6. Avoid sautéed, pan fried, flash-fried, and breaded items.

7. Ask for the gluten-free menu.

8. Avoid cheese sauces like alfredo.

9. Stick with marinara, and red salsa.

10. When ordering broiled fish, ask for it to be dry.

Avoid These Food Traps:

1. Healthy gluten-free granola (not healthy; high in sugar)

2. Gluten-free snacky things like crackers, pretzels, etc. (these = no nutrition)

3. Greek yogurt with fruit (high in sugar)

4. Roasted nuts

5. "Clean-eating" recipes that contain some ingredients that are still high in sugar and too much fat. These are clean cookies, cupcakes, etc., that can contain whole wheat flour with agave nectar, organic cane juice, sugar, or brown sugar

6. Hidden soy ingredients (Read the labels)

7. Veggie burgers (Most contain highly processed vegetables and are fried at restaurants. They can also contain GMO corn or soy products.)

8. Salsas that contain sugar

9. Nut-butters that contain roasted nuts and/or added sugars

For additional recipes, food and snack suggestions as well as TDOS Solutions schedules, please visit www.TheGreenlawReport.com and click on the TDOS Solutions Protocol's. The Greenlaw Report website has a wealth of current information, and we are always adding the latest research and solutions as they become available.

Chapter Nine

More Information on Protein and Amino Acids

I have spent more than a decade learning about high-quality protein sources and how critical protein is to the body. My research allowed me to discover and differentiate between traditional whey proteins versus carefully selected, raw, undenatured whey protein. I also learned how critical protein is for supplying amino acids to the human body. Supplement companies develop their own recipes for straight protein, meal replacement shakes, and amino acid supplements. I have used various meal replacement shakes for years, since my days as a world-class athlete.

For those readers who are interested, this chapter will provide additional in-depth information on the discovery of protein and why it is such an essential part of our diet. It explains a bit more about the role of protein in delivering amino acids to our body, which aid in cell repair and renewal.

"Proteins are the building blocks of life. Through them, genes instruct every physiological change in an organism; determining which cells form which organs; deciding how cells should divide and die. Through them our genes make hair grow, make stomachs digest food, produce tears and saliva."
—**Michael Cordy,** *The Messiah Code*

Protein Delivers Amino Acids to the Body
by Dr. Heinz Reinwald

Proteins may be the single most important molecules that the human body needs. Why is protein so critical to maximize our quality of life potential? Did you know that our body contains more than 20,000 different proteins? If you were to drain all of the fluid out of the human body, you would find that approximately 50 percent of the dry weight of our bodies is protein. But why are proteins so special?

On June 3, 1838, a young Dutch physician and chemist named Gerrit Jan Mulder wrote a letter to his Swedish mentor, Jöns Jacob Berzelius. In a state of great excitement, Mulder revealed an amazing discovery. Young Mulder had been engaged in lively intellectual correspondence with Berzelius for years regarding all matters related to organic chemistry since their first meeting in 1834. In his letter, he told his fatherly friend about a substance he had discovered during research into nitrogenous substances, which he termed "the principle substance of all animals." It did not matter whether the substance was obtained from albumin, fibrin, ovalbumin (egg albumin), or serum albumin from the blood; this substance always had the same basic composition.

On July 10, 1838, Berzelius replied to his young colleague in a letter of equal enthusiasm and with the certainty that research history was being made:

> "The name 'protein' that I am proposing for the organic oxide of fibrin and albumin, I chose to derive from the Greek word PROTEIOS, because it appears to be the

fundamental or primary substance of animal nutrition which plants prepare for herbivores, and who in turn supply it to the carnivores."

Proteins are among the most complex of all nutrients. Like nucleic acids, glycosaminoglycans, and other macromolecules, proteins are not only food but also carry vital information. If there is a type of molecule that can be viewed as the basic building block of living organisms, it would be proteins. Proteins are folded amino acid polymers, each with a specific amino acid sequence. They deliver nutrients and oxygen to the cells, which is critically important for the efficient transportation of the nutritional components that can maximize our quality of life.

Each Protein Has a Unique Identity

Every protein has an individual identity, which helps pinpoint each protein to the species of each amino acid sequence. Proteins are thus important information carriers and form together with nucleic acids, the building blocks of our chromosomes that are made of DNA and proteins. In higher developed life forms, proteins even control neural stimulus and hormonal signals via neuronal secretion.

Proteins are not simply nutrients that the body needs to obtain energy. Unlike fats and carbohydrates, proteins are like small, biological robots that establish and control all living processes through the pre-programmed DNA-RNA code. Without proteins, the genetic information of our genes cannot be used. And, they are the key building blocks of the heart, liver, brain, bones, skin, muscles as well as the organs but also of hormones and neuro-hormones or neuropeptides. When you break it down, life is actually the outcome of a smooth process of protein regeneration, resulting from the correct information shaping all living things.

Protein Controls All Chemical Processes

All chemical processes in living systems are controlled by enzymes, which are in turn protein molecules. Proteins have a fundamental significance as the building blocks of life as well as information carriers like nucleic acids and glycosaminoglycans. In the not so distant future, essential amino acids may become more important for maximizing our quality of life potential than vitamins, minerals, and fatty acids.

Nitrogen Makes the Difference

Like carbohydrates and fats, amino acids consist of hydrogen, oxygen, and carbon. However, as Mulder first demonstrated in the 18th century, they also contain an additional component, nitrogen, which fundamentally differentiates them from carbohydrates and fats. When comparing the molecules, only nitrogen, bound to amino acids, is able to repair and renew tissue. The 70 billion or so cells in our body, hair, skin, and bones, as well as red and white blood cells, the entire immune system, DNA, RNA, as well as enzyme and hormone production depend on the synthesis of protein. They are all constantly being repaired and renewed.

The Role of Amino Acids in the Miracle of Life

Most people do not realize the significance of, or need for, amino acids because they are not aware of the body's massive and perpetual efforts to repair itself. Here are a few figures that give an idea of the extent of the daily maintenance work performed by the body: Between 10 and 50 million cells are broken down and renewed every second, 24 hours a day. Ten thousand instances of repair work required as a result of metabolic activity take place every day in each individual cell. Bone marrow produces 2.5 million red blood cells in a constant manner.

Every four days, the layers of mucous membrane in the stomach are renewed. The majority of the body's white blood cells are replaced within 10 days, and our blood supply is completely renewed every 120 days. Our skin is fully regenerated over 360 days, and the internal organs renew inside 14 months. The biggest detoxifying organ, the liver, is rebuilt eight times over the course of a year. What all this means is that you practically become a different person every seven years!

None of this would be possible without the building blocks of this repair operation, the amino acids that constitute the proteins. Imagine if you crashed your car and the buckled frame straightened itself out within a few weeks, and the body work looked as good as new again. Cell renewal causes precisely the exact same process to occur in the body! Are you beginning to see the critically important role amino acids play in our lives?

Thirty years ago, the discovery of the Human Amino Acid Profile, the optimum amino acid profile for the human diet, was identified by a team of international scientists. This was a major discovery and sensation in nutritional science and medicine.

Proteolysis: The Breakdown of Protein by Enzymes

As we eat protein, our bodies need to extract the individual essential amino acids contained in the food we ingest. In the digestive process, the body breaks down dietary proteins with enzymes (pepsin in the stomach, and proteases like trypsin and chymotrypsin in the small intestine) and then excretes the indigestible part via stool. The first stage of the chemical reaction (or splitting process) occurs in the acidic stomach environment (pH 1.0–1.5), where the protein is split by pepsin and hydrochloric acid into so called peptides—a mixture of short-chain amino acid compounds. This process is called hydrolysis.

Digestion continues in the alkaline environment of the small intestine (> pH 8.0), in which the enzymes trypsin and chymotrypsin break down the protein further. Only these basophilic enzymes in the small intestine are able to split the peptones into amino acids that can be absorbed into the blood through the walls of the small intestine, where they are available to the body to build protein. Both breakdown processes are therefore highly dependent on the pH value surrounding them, meaning they can only work optimally if the milieu is balanced.

In the ideal case of full digestion, the amino acids are able to enter the blood; some of them then follow the anabolic pathway and can be used by the body to build body protein. But some of these amino acids follow the catabolic pathway, which means they are not used as a precursor for body protein synthesis, and they release nitrogen waste and energy. This was not known in nutritional science until the recent discovery by German nutritional scientists and doctors.

THE NUTRITIONAL VALUE OF PROTEIN (NAV)

The Nutritional Value of Protein (NAV), is a scientific measurement, which identifies the percentages of amino acids both utilized and eliminated by the human body. For example, animal proteins average a 30 percent NAV, meaning the body utilizes just 30 percent of the amino acids while the other 70 percent goes to waste, literally turning into toxic waste in the form of urea, creatine, ammonia, and glucose.

This determines the following:

- *Percentage of digestibility*
- *Percentage of the NAV value for body protein synthesis*
- *Amount of energy released (calories)*
- *Percentage of metabolic or nitrogen waste*

Body Protein Synthesis

Together, with the nonessential amino acids produced by the body itself and the aid of transaminase, the eight essential amino acids following the anabolic pathway support the structural foundation of our body as well as all molecules that support life. This process is called body protein synthesis. If the breakdown processes are inadequate because of a lack of acids and pepsin in the stomach, the protein is pushed half-digested into the colon where it is broken down by bacteria, which can place the body under strain, which is evidenced by wind and stools that smell strongly of putrefaction. Mal-digestion or mal-assimilation can therefore lead to a protein deficiency despite a sufficient supply through food.

The latest finding in regards to amino acids and protein metabolism is that amino acids from the digestible part of protein absorbed in the small intestine can follow one of two different metabolic pathways: anabolic (constructive) or catabolic (destructive). This is a unique discovery!

Amino acids that follow the anabolic pathway act as precursors or building blocks for our body protein synthesis; they do not release any energy or nitrogen waste (catabolites).

On the other hand, amino acids that follow the catabolic pathway do not serve as precursors to protein synthesis. As a result, they generate nitrogen catabolites and provide energy (glucose via gluconeogenesis). The following figure illustrates the differences between Anabolic and Catabolic Pathways.

According to this new scientific finding, which replaces our previous understanding that protein always releases energy (4 kcal per gram), we now know that only the part of digestible protein whose amino acids follow the catabolic pathway supplies energy. Amino acids that follow the anabolic pathway, on the other hand, do not generate any energy nor do they generate nitrogen waste. The understanding that one gram of protein provides four large calories is therefore now obsolete. This was determined as far back as 1896 by a researcher named Atwater, by using a calorimeter. At that time, however, nothing was known about protein metabolism.

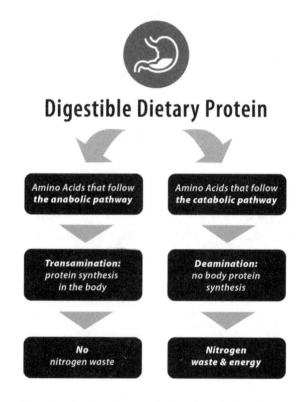

The stages of digestion in anabolic and catabolic pathways

The unbelievable part is that it took more than 100 years before Atwater's work from 1896 was re-examined. Today, we know that there is an inversely proportional link between energy release (catabolic disposal) and the amino acids that follow the anabolic pathway. That is to say, the greater the percentage of amino acids following the anabolic pathway, the lower the number of calories are provided by a particular

protein and vice versa. In other words, while fat (9 kcal) and
carbs (4 kcal) provide constant calories per gram, protein's
calories are not constant. Their calorie output depends on the
specific source of protein.

So what does this mean? The division into two metabolic
pathways, each with a different mechanism of action, means
that not all digestible protein supplied to the body through
food and then split into amino acids can automatically be used
to build new cells. One part, following the catabolic pathway,
is broken down and disposed of as nitrogen waste, which
releases additional energy in the form of calories. The anabolic
pathway is the main function in protein metabolism or body
protein synthesis. With it, all amino acids serve the body by
building new cells, such as organ, muscle, skin, and bone cells,
as well as forming hormones, enzymes, antibodies for the
immune system, and radical scavengers such as glutathione,
which, like cysteine, is a metabolite from the essential amino
acid methionine. It is impossible to generate proper body
protein synthesis by consuming inferior protein or consuming
proteins in which the body is not able to decode the branched
chain amino acids properly. Our best bet? To consume the best
proteins with high concentrations of amino acids.

Essential Amino Acids

Now let's return to the core building blocks of proteins—the
20 proteogenic amino acids. We now know that they are the
ones driven by our genes and they are gene-coded. And we
know that 12 of them are defined as nonessential amino acids
and eight of them are called essential amino acids. This means
that if the body is provided with the eight essential amino acids,
it can make all the proteins it needs, including the other
12 gene-coded ones as well as all the proteins that are non-
coded or non-proteogenic.

Our diet must provide all eight essential amino acids together from one protein source or we will limit our potential for a high quality of life. More important, the lack of any of these may lead to health challenges caused by nutritional deficiency or protein depletion. The nine essential amino acids include:

1. Leucine

2. Phenylalanine

3. Lysine

4. Valine

5. Tryptophan

6. Isoleucine

7. Methionine

8. Threonine

9. Histidine

LEUCINE Braconnot	PHENYLALANINE Schultzw & Barbieri	LYSINE Dreechsel	VALINE Fischer	TRYPTOPHAN Hopkins & Cole	ISOLEUCINE Ehrlich	METHIONINE Muler	THREONINE Rose, McCoy & Meyer
1820	1881	1889	1901	1901	1904	1922	1935

TDOS SOLUTIONS PROVIDER, DR. REINWALD

We are very thankful to Dr. Reinwald for his brilliant explanation of amino acids. Dr. Reinwald is another of our TDOS Solution Providers. Dr. Reinwald is the formulator of My Amino. My Amino as explained by Dr. Reinwald is among the highest quality amino acid supplements in the world.

According to Dr. Reinwald.

In MyAMINO: the unique ratio makes the difference.

MyAMINO is an amino acid formula for protein nutrition with a unique and perfectly balanced amino acid blend in accordance to the specific human amino acid profile. All living organisms, including humans, have a characteristic amino acid profile. MyAMINO provides the eight essential amino acids in a unique ratio for human nutrition. This is how MyAMINO enables a Net Amino Acid Value (NAV) of 99 percent.

This means almost all amino acids can be used as precursors for the body protein synthesis and therefore to build up new cells (anabolic) of the body. Consequently, only 1 percent of the amino acids follow the catabolic pathway and build metabolic waste (nitrogen catabolites like ammonia and energy, (i.e., glucose) compared with soy protein: anabolic 17 percent, catabolic 83 percent. Our organism is only able to build up the body´s own protein optimally when the eight essential amino acids are available in the correct ratio to each other simultaneously. In all other cases, the NAV decreases and the burden of nitrogen catabolites (ammonia) increases. This relieves the liver and the kidneys from an extra burden of nitrogen waste. MyAMINO supplies the highest protein nutritional value compared to other dietary proteins. Thus, it has the lowest amount of metabolic waste like ammonia and energy (i.e., glucose). As it comes in a blend of single, free crystalline amino acids, it doesn't even need proteases to get digested in the small intestine.

This is the way we advise our family, friends, and patients to supplement their daily diets with MyAMINO. This allows the body to have high levels of amino acids utilization with the least amount of nitrogen catabolites and energy i.e. glucose, which for example is part of maximizing our quality of life potential where sugar and carbs should be reduced.

MyAmino can be a great way to infuse the body with super high levels of amino acids, and it can become part of your quality of life system.

Note: The authors of this book receive no financial compensation from the sale of MyAmino. The options expressed are those of Dr. Reinwald and are not intended to treat, diagnose and are not a substitute for medical advice. None of these statements have been evaluated by the FDA.

For additional information on MyAmino please go to
www. www.drreinwald.de/

"Think of the individual amino acids like the pearls on a necklace. A protein is composed of twenty different amino acids that then are put together (utilizing different combinations of the 20 amino acids) in long chain-like structures sometimes containing up to 300 aminos (called branch chain amino acids). If the chain is longer than 100 amino acids, we call them proteins, if it's less, we call them peptides."

—MARCO RUGGIERO, MD

Amino Acids Do Much More Than Build Muscles— They Build Proteins

Amino acids are organic compounds that combine to form proteins. Amino acids and proteins are the building blocks of life. When proteins are digested or broken down, amino acids are what's left. The remaining amino acids assist the body in growing and building muscle as well as breaking down food. The body uses the amino acids that are utilized (extracted from the protein sources we consume) to do a lot more than build muscles. They build the body's human proteins by reassembling the amino acids that have been extracted from the protein source. For example, the body cannot simply take the protein from fish and convert it into the body's own human proteins.

To help explain how this works, here is a simple analogy. There are 26 letters in the roman alphabet, which is shared by several languages. The English word for "book" is "libro" in Italian. Now, imagine that the amino acids contained in proteins from a fish are written in Italian. But unfortunately, the human body only speaks English. If you present to your body the Italian word for book, it has no idea what to do with it. If you separate the letters individually into L I B R O, the body can take the letters B and O from "libro," but it still cannot form the foreign word "book" without the addition of other roman letters from other Italian words. You can see the dilemma in that we are asking our body to reassemble words (human proteins) utilizing the amino acids extracted from a nonhuman protein source (a foreign language).

* * *

Hopefully this chapter gave you a more thorough understanding of why protein and amino acids are so important for your body's overall health. Protein may be the most important food you can consume, which is why the TDOS Solutions include implementing carefully selected, raw, undenatured why protein shakes. Protein transports nutrients and oxygen to our cells and they are the building blocks of the heart, liver, brain, bones, skin, muscles, and organs. The amino acids that constitute proteins help repair millions of our cells every single day. Be sure to incorporate the eight essential amino acids into your diet for optimal wellness.

Notes

Chapter One—Toxicity Interventions

1. Crinnion, Walter J. "Sauna as a Valuable Clinical Tool for Cardiovascular, Autoimmune, Toxicant-induced and Other Chronic Health Problems." *Alternative Medicine Review*, September 2011, 215. Accessed October 28, 2016. Academic OneFile.

2. Gold, Bounous G. "The Biological Activity of Undenatured Dietary Whey Proteins: Role of Glutathione." National Center for Biotechnology Information. Accessed November 06, 2016. http://www.ncbi.nlm.nih.gov/pubmed/1782728

Chapter Two—Nutrient Deficiency Interventions

3. *NFM's Nutrition Science News*, no. 38 (December 1, 1995).

4. Anderson, Arden. "The Root of Good Nutrition." *Organic Connections*, July 2008. www.seaagri.com/docs/arden_anderson.pdf

5. "Thread: New to Raw." The Vegan Forum. Accessed November 06, 2016. http://www.veganforum.com/forums/showthread.php?31928-New-to-raw

6. *Journal of the Medical Association*, June 27, 2012.

Chapter Three—Overweight Interventions

7. "2008 Physical Activity Guidelines for Americans Summary." Accessed October 26, 2016. https://health.gov/paguidelines/guidelines/summary.aspx

8. Gregoire, Carolyn. "How Yoga Changes Your Body, Starting The Day You Begin." *The Huffington Post*. October 28, 2013. Accessed November 06, 2016. http://www.huffingtonpost.com/2013/10/28/body-on yoga_n_4109595.html

Chapter Four—Stress Interventions

9. Stroebel, Charles, *The Quieting Reflex*, Berkely, 1985.

10. Pawar, Vinod S., and Hugar Shivakumar. "A Current Status of Adaptogens: Natural Remedy to Stress." *Asian Pacific Journal of Tropical Disease* 2 (2012). doi:10.1016/s2222-1808(12)60207-2.

Chapter Six—Sustaining Your Health Momentum

11. Thyer, Lynda, Emma Ward, Rodney Smith, Maria Fiore, Stefano Magherini, Jacopo Branca, Gabriele Morucci, Massimo Gulisano, Marco Ruggiero, and Stefania Pacini. "A Novel Role for a Major Component of the Vitamin D Axis: Vitamin D Binding Protein-Derived Macrophage Activating Factor Induces Human Breast Cancer Cell Apoptosis through Stimulation of Macrophages." *Nutrients* 5, no. 7 (2013): 2577-589. doi:10.3390/nu5072577.

Bibliography

Acheson, K. et al. (2011). Protein choices targeting thermogenesis and metabolism. *The American Journal of Clinical Nutrition*, Vol. 93 No. 3 pp. 525-534.

Baillie-Hamilton, P. (2005). *Toxic Overload*. New York: Avery.

Beach, R. (1936). *Modern Miracle Men*. Washington, D.C.: U.S. Government Printing Office.

Campbell, W. et al. (2001). The recommended dietary allowance for protein may not be adequate for older people to maintain skeletal muscle. *Journal of Gerontology: Biological Sciences*, Vol. 56, Issue 6; pp. M373-M380.

Colgan, M. (2001). *The New Power Program: Protocols for Maximum Strength*. Apple Publishing Co.

Dangin, M. et al. (2001). The digestion rate of protein is an independent regulating factor of postprandial protein retention. *Am J Physiol Endocrinol Metab.*, Feb;280(2):E340-8.

Edwardes, C. (2003, September 14). Mr Banting's Old Diet Revolution. *The Telegraph*. London.

Encyclopædia Britannica. (2012). Retrieved July 30, 2012, from http://www.britannica.com/EBchecked/topic/90141/calorie

Enig, M. (1995). *Trans Fatty Acids in the Food Supply: A Comprehensive Report Covering 60 Years of Research*. Silver Spring, MD: Enig Associates, Inc.

Enig, M. (2000). *Know Your Fats: The Complete Primer for Understanding the Nutrition of Fats, Oils and Cholesterol*. Silver Spring, MD: Bethesda Press.

Enig, M.; Fallon, S. (1999). *Nourishing Traditions*. Washington, D.C.: New Trends Publishing.

Environmental Working Group. (2005, July 14). Study Finds Industrial Pollution Begins in the Womb. *News Release*. Washington, D.C.

EPA, U. (1990). *The National Human Adipose Tissue Survey*.

Fallon, S. (1996). Tripping Lightly Down the Prostaglandin Pathways. *Price-Pottenger Nutrition Foundation Health Journal*, 20:3:5-8.

Fallon, S. (2001). *Nourishing Traditions.* Washington, D.C.: New Trends Publishing.

Felton, C. et al. (1994). Dietary polyunsaturated fatty acids and compositions of human aortic plaque. *Lancet,* 344:1195-1196.

Finkelstein, E. (2012). Obesity and Severe Obesity Forecasts through 2030. *American Journal of Preventive Medicine,* Vol. 42, Issue 6, Pages 563-570.

Foxcroft, L. (2011). *Calories & Corsets: A History of Dieting Over 2000 Years.* London: Profile Books.

Gruber, B. (2002, May 25). *The History of Diets and Dieting.* Retrieved from CarbSmart: http://www.carbsmart.com/historydiets.html

Grun, F., & Blumberg, B. (2006). Environmental Obesogens: Organotins and Endocrine Disruption via Nuclear Receptor Signaling. *Endocrinology,* Vol. 147 No. 6 s50-s55.

Harper, D. (2012). Doctor of Osteopathy

Holtcamp, W. (2012). Obesogens: An Environmental Link to Obesity. *Environmental Health Perspective,* 120:a62-a68.

Houlihan, J., Kropp, T., Wiles, R., Gray, S., & Campbell, C. (2005). *Body Burden: The Pollution in Newborns.* Environmental Working Group.

Hyman, M. (2009). *The Ultra Mind Solution.* New York: Scribner.

Karnani, M. et al. (2011). Activation of Central Orexin/Hypocretin Neurons by Dietary Amino Acids. *Neuron,* 72: 616-629.

Kim, J; Li, Y; Watkins, B. (2011). Endocannabinoid signaling and energy metabolism: a target for dietary intervention. *Nutrition,* June 27 (6):624-32.

Lassek, W.; Gaulin, S. (2012). *Why Women Need Fat.* New York: Hudson Street Press.

Lasserre, M. et al. (1985). Effects of different dietary intake of essential fatty acids on C20:3 omega 6 and C20:4 omega 6 serum levels in human adults. *Lipids,* Apr;20(4):227-33.

Mann, T. et al. (2007, April). Medicare's Search for Effective Obesity Treatments: Diets Are Not the Answer. *American Psychologist,* pp. Vol. 62, No. 3, 220–233.

Miller, D. (2011). Retrieved from www.lewrockwell.com: http://www.lewrockwell.com/miller/miller38.1.html

National Institutes of Health. (2009, March 16). Study Helps Unravel Mysteries of Brain's Endocannabinoid System. U.S. Department of Health and Human Services.

Ogden, C.; Carroll, M. (2010). *Prevalence of Overweight, Obesity, and Extreme Obesity Among Adults: United States, Trends 1960–1962 Through 2007–2008.* Centers for Disease Control and Prevention.

Pennings, B. et al. (2011, May). Whey protein stimulates postprandial muscle protein accretion more effectively than do casein and casein hydrolysate in older men. *The American Journal of Clinical Nutrition,* pp. 93(5):997-1005.

Perrine, S. (2010). *The New American Diet.* Rodale Inc.

Peters, L. H. (1918). *Diet and Health: With Key to The Calories.* Chicago: The Reilly & Lee Co.

Pimentel, D. L. (1986). *Pesticides: Amounts Applied and Amounts Reaching Pests.* American Institute of Biological Sciences.

Pinckney, E. et al. (1973). *The Cholesterol Controversy.* Los Angeles: Sherbourne Press.

Pollan, M. (2006). *The Omnivore's Dilemma.* New York: The Penguin Press.

Schauss, M. (2008). *Achieving Victory Over a Toxic World.* Bloomington, IN: Author House.

Stitt, P. (1982). *Beating the Food Giants.* Natural Press.

STOP Obesity Alliance Research Team. (2010). *Improving Obesity Management in.* Washington, D.C.: The George Washington University School of Public Health and Health Services.

The Endocrine Society. (2009). *Endocrine-Disrupting Chemicals.* Chevy Chase, MD.

USDA. (2011). *Sugar and Sweeteners Outlook, No. (SSSM-273).* Washington, D.C.: U.S. Department of Agriculture.

Valero-Garrido, D. et al. (1990). Influence of Dietary Fat on the Lipid Composition of Perirenal Adipose Tissue in Rats. *Annals of Nutrition and Metabolism,* 34:327-332.

vom Saal, F. et al. (2012). The estrogenic endocrine disrupting chemical bisphenol A (BPA) and obesity. *Molecular and Cellular Endocrinology,* 354: 74-84.

Weinberg, B., & Bealer, B. (2001). *The World of Caffeine: The Science and Culture of the World's Most Popular Drug.* New York: Routledge.

Wilkinson, A. (1995, June 5). Oh, What A Tangled Web. *The New Yorker,* p. 34.

Wilson, L. (2011). *Selenium: A Critical Mineral for Health and Healing.* Prescott, AZ: Center for Development.

Index

O

P

About the Authors

Peter Greenlaw has conducted more than 1,500 lectures around the world on health topics and the ideas he presents in this book. He has been the featured speaker at the Autism One conferences in 2014 and 2015, a frequent speaker at the CEO Club of New York City, and a guest on many television programs in such cities as Washington, DC, Los Angeles, San Francisco, Portland, and Kansas City. Greenlaws first TV show, *The New Health Conversation* aired on Rocky Mountain PBS, where he introduced a fresh approach to health, diet, nutrition and TDOS. He will be the central figure in an upcoming television pilot being filmed by award-winning director Douglas Freel titled *The Greenlaw Report*™.

Nicholas Messina, MD, became a board-certified family physician in 1985. He was a solo practitioner from 1985-1994. He formed a group family practice in 1994. During this time, Dr. Messina was the Deputy Director of Family Practice for St. Joseph Hospital in Stamford, Connecticut, and he served on several hospital committees. In 1997 he became the Medical Director for a Complementary Wellness Center in Norwalk, Connecticut. In 1999 he became the medical director for an Independent Clinical Research Facility in Mesa, Arizona. He has been the Principal Investigator on numerous clinical trials involving many of the Fortune 500 Pharmaceutical companies. The trials included medications for arthritis, diabetes, depression, obesity, chronic pain, generalized anxiety. and other conditions. He also served as the Vice Chairman of the Board for an Independent Ethics Committee (IRB), overseeing pharmaceutical research to ensure sound scientific design and subject safety. He has been published in peer reviewed medical journals and has written articles on health related issues for several magazines He currently resides in Mesa, Arizona and does private consulting for the Healthcare, Pharmaceutical, and Financial industries.

Drew Greenlaw graduated from the University of Colorado with a degree in English. He currently lives in Colorado with his wife and three kids. Drew started working with his father, Peter, eight years ago. The two collaborated on a research project to build a case against toxins and their effects on the human body. This early research would set the stage for the discovery of the TDOS Syndrome®. Drew continues to work behind the scenes on research and development for the new show *The Greenlaw Report*™, as well as their website www.PeterGreenlaw.com. The intention of both the show and website are to provide additional solutions as well as solution providers to further help and educate people on the current state of health and wellness.